BODY EN

Books available from the same author in the series
By Appointment Only:

Stress and Nervous Disorders (fifth impression)

Multiple Sclerosis (second impression)

Traditional Home and Herbal Remedies (third impression)

Arthritis, Rheumatism and Psoriasis (fourth impression)

Do Miracles Exist?

Neck and Back Problems (fourth impression)

Migraine and Epilepsy (second impression)

Cancer and Leukaemia

Viruses, Allergies and the Immune System (second impression)

Realistic Weight Control

Who's Next?

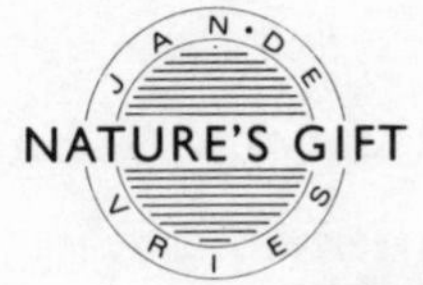

Body Energy

JAN DE VRIES

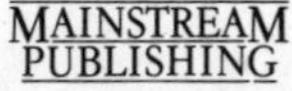

Reprinted 1992

First published in 1989 by
MAINSTREAM PUBLISHING CO. (EDINBURGH) LTD.
7 Albany Street
Edinburgh EH1 3UG

ISBN 1 85158 262 2 (cloth)
ISBN 1 85158 267 3 (paper)

British Library Cataloguing in Publication Data
Vries, Jan de, 1943—
Body energy
1. Man. Health. Improvement
I. Title
613

ISBN 1-85158-262-2
ISBN 1-85158-267-3 pbk

Typeset in 10½/12½ Palatino.
Reproduced from disc by Polyprint,
48 Pleasance, Edinburgh, EH8 9TJ.

Printed in Great Britain by Billing & Sons, Worcester.

This book is dedicated to Leonard J. Allan DO, ND, DrAc., who freely presented me with his findings from years of research into energy and from whom I have learned so much.

The natural healing force within each one of us is the greatest force in getting well.

Hippocrates

Contents

1

Universal Energy

STANDING ON THE TOP of a hill overlooking the majestic scenery of the Clyde coast and gazing at the awe-inspiring valley in which stands Culzean Castle, I contemplated the mysterious ground on which I found myself yet again. Although I have travelled the world and have seen many inexplicable phenomena, curiosity repeatedly draws me back to this particular spot. It is called Croy Brae, or, to most people from the west coast of Scotland, the "Electric Brae".

I stood there contemplating for some time and when I looked around I saw, as usual, some children rolling balls up the Brae. They placed them on the slope and, on letting go, they watched their balls roll *up* the hill! Whenever I am there, I watch the faces of the people in the cars that glide silently past. Most drivers put their cars in neutral, release the handbrake and marvel at the sensation of being drawn up the Brae as if by magic. Instead of rolling backwards, as would be expected, they find themselves miraculously carried to the summit of the hill.

I decided to call in the help of a friend of mine whom I regard as the best person to advise me on the mysteries relating to the subject of energy. The phenomenon I have just described is usually explained away as an optical illusion. When I think back to my schooldays, however, I remember learning the easy definition of an optical illusion being a shape, a size or distance of an object that is misperceived because of the influence of the immediate surroundings. Even so, for over twenty years I had accepted the theory that this was the most likely explanation for what occurs at the Electric Brae, though possibly with a certain measure of doubt.

I duly asked my friend to come over and visit the place with me. After he had used his surveyor's level, he told me that part of the Brae does indeed fall as the road turns the corner and passes the sign-post. From that point on, the road rises slightly at a rate of four feet in every hundred yards. As a result of the topography of the surrounding fields sloping towards the sea, an illusion is created that the road continues to fall.

With a proper survey of the road, using a theodolite, it would be possible to quantify the fall in levels of the road to fractions of an inch and so calculate the levels in the fields causing the illusion. However, after having surveyed the area geologically, my friend was surprised to see that a very strong electro-magnetic field was present, covering the entire stretch of the roadway designated as the Electric Brae. Therefore, although it was partially true that the Brae is an optical illusion, as I had expected, there was more to it. A study of the rock formation suggests that a wide band of low-level magnetite lies below the area. Similar wide bands of magnetite rock, i.e. black iron oxide, are not uncommon in many parts of the world and research into reported earthquakes point to inexplicable geophysical phenomena occurring in such areas.

My friend checked out the herd record book of a local farmer to determine when and where animals might have died from unknown causes. Sometimes, for example, spontaneous combustion takes place in haystacks and this is another recognised phenomenon in areas of magnetite rock. In the research my friend has done into these fires, it has been shown that the date, time and location of their occurrence can be established precisely according to a predictive survey. Measurements between fire grounds also allow calculations to be carried out to determine certain causative elements.

On further investigation of the Electric Brae, my friend discovered a strong presence of both magnetite and germanium in conflict under this particular hill. This indicated the existence of an energy disturbance, which I felt compelled to study further.

As a doctor of acupuncture I am greatly involved with, and have a strong interest in, energy fields. It is a fact that the body is one large field of energy and therefore I make the most of every opportunity to study energy. Yet I also know that our present knowledge of energy constitutes only a fraction of what still remains to be learned about it. One thing, however, is without doubt, and that is that whenever we are able to balance energy, we are more than halfway towards effecting a recovery from certain illnesses and diseases. And that is what this book is all about. I look upon it as a challenge to find the normal energy actions for things that have been labelled as mysterious or magical, and which often prove to be basically a matter of energy balancing. The theory that disease cannot exist in a balanced energy field is all too true and in my work I have set out to prove that fact during the past thirty years or so that I have been in practice.

Through all my observations I have come to believe that in disease or illness the symptoms manifest themselves as changes in the body. I also firmly believe that such symptoms exist as a field of energy and can be shown as such with the use of certain techniques. Regardless of whether that field of energy sends negative or positive impulses, the body organs do receive energy from each other. All too often we see that where there is a blockage of energy, the healthy organs grow weaker and energy will not be transmitted from the diseased organs. Very often other illnesses will then occur. This tends to happen in stages, as if it were a reaction to a deposit of accumulated toxins or excretions. This process becomes apparent as a result of accidents, operations, depressions, degeneration or any other interference in the energy flow. Very often, therefore, after interviewing a patient I will look for signs as to where the energy might be disturbed. Like all living creatures, man lives in an electro-magnetic environment from which nothing can be isolated.

Good health is totally dependent on a good energy balance and an unhindered flow of energy that follows the paths of the meridians. Energy flows through the body in a circle, thus making the beginning and the end of each body part very important. Since energy can never flow in one direction only, it follows that the laws of polarity between energy and cells become relevant. Hundreds of factors can influence an interference in this system.

Some time ago I was consulted by a priest who complained of sudden fierce pains in the sigmoid area. He had consulted every doctor and specialist he could think of, but his problems persisted. When he came to me I found that the solution was simple. I suspected a blockage in his energy flow and narrowed down the cause of this to dental amalgam. After the priest's amalgam fillings had been replaced with composite fillings, I managed to restore the energy flow with very little effort, for which he was extremely grateful.

Energy can be restored in many ways, such as improved dietary management, specific remedies, acupuncture or manipulation. To name but a few reasons for a disturbance in the energy balance, we need look no further than lack of exercise, stress, overwork, a poor diet, a virus or toxic conditions. When one's energy is out of balance, one's health is affected, hence the importance of knowing how to influence this electro-magnetic field of energy in order to restore the energy flow.

Considering the above, it is more easily understood why nowadays we seem to be more prone to such influences as viruses and allergies, because of the way they disturb the energy flow. Positive energy can promote particular forms of life, but a balance between negative and positive energy is also essential. If that balance is missing and there is a loss of energy, we cannot fight off disease.

Atmospheric influences cause great problems in this respect, as control of the hydrogen ion is most important for the chemical action that takes place in the human body. Every cell in our body is part of the body's electric field and we are fortunate in that we are now able to measure the energy field in the body. In a diseased body, this can be measured using the latest Vincent methods; in this way cancer, for example, can be detected in the very early stages. As always, when the immune system is weakened, the body is unable to cope with bacteria and viruses, and ill health will result. If the energy in the body is balanced, the immune system functions more effectively and we need not fear ill health.

Each disease has a specific energy pattern and through that pattern we know what to expect and what can be done to overcome that particular condition. As I have mentioned already, energy in the human body can easily be disturbed by seemingly insignificant factors. When I have noticed that the immune system of a patient is affected because of unbalanced energy, I have sometimes traced factors that appear relatively innocent, and yet play a strong role in dete[illegible]ining the patient's state of health. The energy flow can [illegible] because we, possibly unwittingly, have inte[illegible]dy energies and we should never fail to [illegible] we obey the laws of nature, we also ob[illegible]rgy.

[illegible]es when I graduated, I saw the first si[illegible]ngers. We then witnessed the explosion o[illegible]nquillisers and other "wonderful" drugs. [illegible]alise at the time that even though these [illegible] appear to be our allies and certainly act to our *immediate* advantage, equally often they serve as our enemies in that they interfere with the natural energy flow. As such, they lower the efficiency of the immune system and create alternative problems to the ones they were intended to solve.

We must learn to listen to our body and perhaps ask ourselves where we could have gone wrong. There is no need to be paranoid about this, but it is wise to stop and listen to our body language, as the body does send out messages. If we can learn to interpret these messages to our advantage, the causative conditions can then be discovered more easily. Unfortunately, in today's society this is more essential than ever before. The great gift of magnetic energy is universal and when we come to appreciate that everything in this world, including space, has its own magnetic energy, we will become more closely connected to the entire universe.

It was in the year 1720 that Steven Grey discovered electricity. The medical world had long been aware that there existed an underlying source of all body functions, without exactly being able to refer to electricity as such. Now we know that electricity is composed of electrons and protons, and that even the smallest particles exist in the physical plane. Hence the fact that hydrogen ions are a key in the answer to our present problems concerning immunity. All disease starts with energy loss and all health and disease depends on how the body handles the hydrogen ion balance. Many diseases become apparent when there is an imbalance in the acid/alkaline levels. Fortunately, once such problems have been detected we know of many methods with which such conditions can be brought under control again.

In my book *Viruses, Allergies and the Immune System* I have already stressed how important it is that we keep the environment clean, as so many aspects resulting from modern advances in technology have an atmospheric influence on this balance. The little electrical currents which govern the life of humans, animals, plants and all living systems, depend on energy which is controlled by the hydrogen ion balance and it is gratifying to know that we have learned to re-establish a balance once it has been lost.

Quite some time ago now, I visited a witch doctor in a remote part of Africa. There I witnessed this man trying, with every form of mysticism known to him, to cure a badly arthritic man. It was absolutely unheard of for a white man to touch a native, but through my interpreter I acquired certain information relating to the patient's condition. I offered some suggestions and finally I was allowed to place some zinc and copper magnets on specific acupuncture points. I had noticed that the body posture of the patient, who was almost crippled, was totally out of alignment and therefore I chose the acupuncture points that relate to the south and north poles.

With the help of the magnets, I indeed succeeded in correcting the imbalance. The witch doctor then desperately sought to obtain for himself the magnets that had achieved such remarkable results. No doubt he intended to add them to his bag of tricks, but without the necessary knowledge of the specific acupuncture points to restore balance, they would do him little good!

By studying energy, we soon realise that the timing of the treatment is as important as the way in which the energy is directed, i.e. from the north and south poles towards each particular area in the body.

A number of eminent scientists and physicians have expressed their opinion on the fields of energy in the human body. It was the great Max Gerson who said: "I am convinced that the problem of chronic disease is not one of biochemistry; rather it is produced by deeper lying forces which cause the deficiencies of energy." And my friend Dr Leonard Allan maintained that the body, which is an extension of the earth, has three fields: the emotional-electric field, the mental electric-magnetic field and the electrical magnetic field.

The word 'disease' means dis-ease, i.e. a lack of ease, harmony or well-being. 'Emotion' means a moving out of energy. The energy fields in the body have to be normalised or balanced before a patient's disease or symptoms can be corrected. I sometimes think that perhaps we have moved too far away from nature and perhaps we see things too scientifically. Yet, if only we took the trouble to ask ourselves where and why the energy is disturbed, we could see it corrected. We have the knowledge and tools to restore energy, and by doing so we can again experience the great wonder of creation and its universal energy.

These were more or less my thoughts when I was sitting near the Electric Brae. I also thought of the other thousands of visitors who in the years to come may pause there for a moment to look out over the Firth of Clyde and admire the grandeur of the massifs of Goat Fell and other mountains on Arran shimmering in the distance, where the volcanic granite bulk of Ailsa Craig stands as a gateway, shining in the morning sun. Only a few people would perhaps understand one of nature's great wonders in this little area of Croy Brae. Some may stop to ask a local about this phenomenon and may be treated to some of the tales of the supernatural and other weird stories that have been handed down for generations. After all, the hero of Robert Burns' poem "Tam o' Shanter" came from a farm in the vicinity of the Electric Brae.

Is there a logical explanation for the feeling of unease experienced when intense static energy makes a person's hair stand on end? Similarly, it is possible that vibrations may cause a certain unease when standing on this rocky formation with its inherent electro-magnetic energy. The disturbance or fault line in this part of the country is referred to in the archives together with data concerning inexplicable geophysical phenomena, indicating a time/distance basis of the electro-magnetic energy being emitted from its underground power.

Many years ago, the Yugoslavian engineer and inventor Tesla illustrated the power of such sub-strata energy. Today, research has confirmed that this energy, now named "geopathic stress", affects many forms of matter, including any person who is below a certain level of health. The understanding of this low-level electro-magnetic energy has led to many seemingly inexplicable natural phenomena being scientifically explained, including spontaneous combustion, seismical disease or chemical instability. Even the vast atomic periodic table of organic and inorganic elements can now be quantified in terms of time, distance, colour and tonal harmony and the wave frequency of an electro-magnetic energy.

On that day, as I made ready to leave this fascinating spot at the Electric Brae, I looked all around me and pondered on the enormous cosmic energy. I looked upwards and could not help but think of that wonderful biblical quotation:

> When I look at the sky which You have made, at the moon and the stars which You have set in those places, what is man that You think of him, mere man that You care for him?

2

Innate Energy

I AM FREQUENTLY asked for my opinion on the future of medicine and I always say that to my way of thinking the key to that lies in energy. Within the subject of energy I have come to the conclusion that innate energy is something quite special. Quite a few years ago now, I was in the United States and was invited to attend a seminar at which a lecturer was due to speak on the subject of innate energy. I must admit that I was intrigued by this at the time. I considered "innate energy" to be a rather unusual expression, but only when I sat down to listen to this lecture did I understand what this phrase referred to. Like this lecturer, I too have discovered over the years that innate energy in man is often inexplicable, as it works in mysterious ways.

The lecturer claimed that by the use of his thumbs only, he was able to restore energy. By studying the law of motion he had learned how the positive and negative energy flow could be used to control cause and effect.

Man expresses energy with every tick of the clock — even by inhalation. Every inhalation must be followed by exhalation or the correct sequence of the principle is broken. In their efforts to restore harmony the importance of this innate energy was known to the early acupuncturists practising so many centuries ago. Man's energy within himself, and its structural balance with the earth's gravity and the finer fields of nature's energy, should be understood by man as part of the universe in which he is placed.

We know that every molecule and atom in the universe — animate or inanimate — is in constant vibration. Each mineral and each life cell in man or any animal vibrates and has its own frequency and wavelength. We have also come to the conclusion that energy vibration, or cosmic energy vibration, has a profound influence on our lives. We are in constant contact with cosmic forces and these energies are extremely powerful. The complete identity of man consists of body, mind and soul. Each human body cell is composed of atoms and has a nucleus of solar electricity which dominates its magnetic force. This force is not easily understood and sometimes reacts in a totally different manner to what we may have expected.

We may have the ability to stimulate or to subdue energies in the body, but we do not always receive the right indications as to whether the energies that exist in every organ, tissue, muscle or bone are in direct or indirect contact with the human body. Early acupuncturists were aware of this centuries ago and realised that by using needles on certain energy points, endorphins and encephalins could be released to diminish pain. In the same way, however, they could also harmonise energy and enhance the innate energy of man, that energy for which we have no satisfactory explanation, as the phrase itself indicates, "innate energy", i.e. something that exists naturally rather than an acquired attribute.

Occasionally, we experience how this innate energy may respond to being pointed in the right direction in a way which is totally beyond our expectations. This happened to me with a Multiple Sclerosis patient who had been reduced to life in a wheelchair. After I had used certain acupuncture energy points, this patient fully recovered the use of her legs. Perhaps I had chosen an energy point that was specific to this individual, but the proof was there to be seen. The innate energy had thus been allowed to flow freely through this patient's legs and once her muscles had regained their strength she was able to walk again.

Energy centres exist on the surface of the skin and through these centres one can endeavour to heal or stimulate these inherent or innate universal energies. This can be done with needles; it can be done with the hands; or it can be done with a simple touch — as we will see in later chapters of this book.

Cosmic power is *the* power of the universe and it is of the utmost importance that a balance of this energy in the human body is retained. Whether or not we can scientifically explain this fact is of secondary importance to the knowledge that vibrations cause energy. Vibrations are soaked up in the same way as a sponge absorbs water and, no matter how careful we are, our conscious system will accept vibration, just as our body accepts the food that enters our stomach. Vibration in a negative sense can lead to an imbalance in innate energy. In my book *Do Miracles Exist?* I have mentioned several such examples.

You may be surprised to learn that even our thoughts can alter the energy flow and I have sometimes proved this to sceptics with the help of Kirlian photography. Encourage a patient to think a positive thought and then take a photograph of the energy outflow. Then compare this picture to a photograph taken after a negative thought and you will see how disarranged and disturbed the energy flow has become. With respect to this subject it is worth knowing that our thought faculties are divided into three separate parts: objective, subjective and subconscious. Our thinking is transferred from the universal mind to three divisions of our brain. Our thoughts, actions and deeds depend greatly upon the action of our conscious system — upon our brain. If the organisms of the body are not functioning properly, they interfere with the conscious system of our brain, thus causing heavy and sluggish thinking. In order to have a clear brain, then, we need clear action. We must make sure that the body is functioning properly, and free from aches and pains. Our body, soul and spirit should be in good balance. Unfortunately, this is the case with only a few of us.

Energy vibration positively helps the innate energy to flow more freely and without interruption. All life is energy; all energy is vibration and vibration, in turn, is energy. These are principal facts in the universe. Every vibration is a movement of something in a certain direction at a certain rate. Therefore, if there is a disturbance in our innate energy flow, even a touch in the right place can solve certain real problems. Tissue vibration can cause the subconscious mind to make all the tissues of the body subject to similar vibrations.

This constitutes not only a practical approach to the patient, it is a mechanical stimulus to the patient's body energy as a field of energy. How easily this innate energy can be disturbed has recently become apparent from the results of tests on people who spend too much time sitting in front of a word processor or a computer screen. It is now a recognised fact that doing so can cause great disruption to the balance of energy in the human body.

We also see this effect in people who live near power stations and, again, recent research has indicated that other forms of radiation, such as microwaves or radio frequencies, can be just as dangerous. I myself have conducted tests on television addicts to determine how their energy output differs before and after a spell in front of the screen. It is important that we are aware of the risks of such influences, especially for those whose work involves exposure to monitor screens on a regular basis. Precautionary measures exist and guidelines have been laid down concerning these which one would be wise to adhere to.

If you happen to fall into this category, make sure, for example, that you undergo ophthalmic tests at frequent intervals, that a record is kept of the machines you have used and that you take advantage of the recommended recovery periods and protective radiation shields available.

For sensitive individuals, a Voll test, a Vega test, or a Compruton test are invaluable for measuring the differences in body energy fields in such cases. It is most important that you are fully aware of the possible risks attached to such working conditions.

An imbalanced energy flow that affects the innate energy can be corrected. We know that the body is not perfect and we also know that the environment we live in today requires us to pay more attention to such factors than was previously the case.

By touching or massaging the body tissue of muscles, we can coax the muscles into fulfilling their original functions. We can measure their strengths and their weaknesses. We can learn to locate an acupuncture point and massage a painful area therapeutically, either clockwise, anticlockwise, in circular movements or sideways. For this we can either use one, two or more fingers, or place one or two hands partly over the painful or diseased area. In later chapters of this book you will read about muscle testing and how we can improve the energy flow with such simple methods as I have mentioned above. However, in order to understand our body language, we have first to recognise what is happening. In this respect I can recommend the excellent book *Touch for Health*, written by John F. Thie, from which we can learn how to restore these natural energies.

If you need further convincing, try out the following simple test with a friend or a member of the family. Ask your partner to stand upright facing towards you, with his right arm relaxed at his side and left arm held straight out, parallel to the floor. Place your left hand on his right shoulder and with your right hand grip his extended arm just above the wrist. Tell him that you are going to push on his arm while he tries to resist with all his strength. Push down his arm quickly and firmly, just hard enough to feel the spring, and in nearly every case the muscle will hold firm.

For the second part of the test, do one of the following things: tell him to think about pressure at work; suggest that he looks at a neon lamp or that he thinks of something he finds unpleasant. This time you will most likely find that he will then be unable to resist the pressure on his arm. This exercise is just one simple way of testing how certain influences will affect our innate energy. It also serves to prove that we tend to underestimate the power of innate energy.

You may appreciate the story of the violinist who had the misfortune to become a victim of an energy disturbance. During a recital, one of the strings of his violin suddenly snapped, immediately followed by a second string. He then became aware of a pain in his right arm and subsequently lost the use of this arm. After extensive tests, specialists informed him that he was suffering from Multiple Sclerosis. These circumstances forced him to give up his work and signalled the end of his musical career.

It was not till later that the true cause of this unfortunate incident became known. The site where this turn of events took place was checked out and it was found that the energy flow was badly disturbed. It was then learned that there had been an earthquake in that particular area a considerable time ago. The innate energy in the area was still affected by this natural disaster; in fact it appeared to be permanently disturbed at that particular geographical point. The violinist had become the victim of this disturbance in the energy flow.

In the case of another patient diagnosed as having Multiple Sclerosis, it was discovered that in the house where he lived, there had been two earlier occupants who had received the same diagnosis. Again, this patient's complaint was subsequently ascribed to an energy disruption. The serious effects on the sympathetic nervous system had disturbed the innate energy to such an extent that the people involved completely lost the power in their arms and legs. From these case histories let us learn a lesson on the necessity of harmonious energy. And let us not forget that negative or positive vibrations can lead to imbalances that are often hard to detect.

You have now read some of the reasons for my statement that the future of medicine lies in energy, or, to be more precise, in the balance of energy. We do not know all there is to know about energy, but we will increase our knowledge as we proceed. At present, at least we are aware of the healing powers of cosmic energy and understand that it contains three aspects, i.e. physical, mental and emotional. We also know already of various methods that can be used to balance innate energy and several forms of treatment to this effect have been adopted in the field of complementary medicine, for example, acupuncture, osteopathy, reflexology and colour therapy. Successful treatment could merely involve applying a simple touch or a small magnet, if this is placed in the right position. In addition, there are many more methods that can be used, such as dietary management, natural herb remedies, homoeopathy, music and sound therapy, to name but a few.

The existence of innate energy can be scientifically proven. It can also be measured in several ways and here Kirlian photography can be used very successfully.

Apart from investigating the life energy of plants, food, seeds, etc., Kirlian photography can be used in the following ways:

(a) to assist in the process of familiarisation and diagnosis when the patient is seen for the first time;
(b) to observe the effects of a treatment or therapy. It is of particular relevance when the patient presents unclear or ambiguous symptoms or does not respond to treatment over a period of time. Specifically, the method can highlight the following features:
—the level of energy patterns of degeneration
—the balance between the two sides of the body (yin and yang)
—the nature and extent of any emotional problems
—the level of physical tension

—the extent of psychological withdrawal
—the general stability of personality
—an organic imbalance (correlating with reflexology and acupuncture)
—the degree of the patient's resistance to treatment
—the overall condition of the spine and associated weaknesses.

Remember the words of William Shakespeare:

> There are more things in Heaven and Earth, Horatio,
> Than are dreamt of in your philosophy.
>
> (*Hamlet*)

3

Mind Energy

"IF YOU DON'T want trouble, don't think it and don't say it. Words are thoughts with a birth certificate. Once said, they are firmly recorded."

This is a quote from the American author R. D. Granville and there is a lot of wisdom and truth in these words. On the whole, we fail to recognise energy from the mind or energy in our thoughts for its capabilities. However, logic dictates that one single idea or initial thought can result in a course of action that can possibly change our lives, and that one single thought can produce either a positive or negative reaction. Mind energy can be compared to electrical impulses in the mind that can result in great physical energy; therefore the saying "As man thinketh, so shall he be", is positively true.

All rational human beings act according to their thoughts and it therefore follows that their actions are a product of those thoughts. This, of course, excludes cases of accident and trauma. It is, then, a rational progression to assume that disease is a product of thought and that the mind is stronger than the body. In my practice I have frequently witnessed how patients have been able to cure themselves through the application of positive mind energy. The phrase "mind over matter" indicates replacing negative thoughts by positive thoughts. Sometimes that process is half the battle. From the thousands of patients I have seen and treated, I have also learned that when their thoughts were positive, the energy balance would be restored far more quickly. In such cases I have seen apparently miraculous recoveries and in my book *Do Miracles Exist?* I have related several such instances of patients who have cured themselves by thinking positively. It is, then, true that patients can discipline their thinking in order to reverse the negative influences on their health.

In a wonderful book, *The Computer and the Brain,* by Dr John van Newman, I read that the human brain possesses the attributes of both the analogue and the digital computer. How we use these attributes is up to ourselves. It is claimed that science has confirmed that every human being has been engineered for success and that every human being has access to that great power within himself. However, the conscious mind, through its capacity to judge in terms of negative assessment, can also decide to criticise the physical self. Physiological conditions may then occur because the mental cells can be affected by negative thoughts, the body consciousness may choose to accept this negative judgement. It could therefore follow that anger, stress, nervous anxiety, doubt, or any negative thought may cause an energy imbalance.

The physical cell has a counterpart which is a cellular twin possessing a subtle form of energy which works in physical and non-physical conjunction so that each cell knows what its course of activity and destination is. Seven kinds of energy exist, which are basic points to set the wheel of energy in motion with its degrees of transmutation. It is a great miracle to stretch the mind to see what it is capable of and that the cells will rebel if certain energy patterns in our mind and thinking are not being utilised. The body needs to transmute and transmutation is done on a regular basis.

In my book *Cancer and Leukaemia* you can read about instances where mind, thought and vibration can prove harmful if positive thinking is not applied to draw out the beneficial effects of a particular influence. With this in mind, I must tell you about an experience that made a great impression on me at the time, and although it happened when I was still quite young, I have never forgotten it.

I must have been around the age of ten or twelve, when our neighbour's daughter was diagnosed as being terminally ill with cancer. Her parents had made up a bed for her in front of the window so that she would be able to look out and see what was going on outside. Everyone who passed by would wave to her. She spent a lot of time there, because the deterioration in her condition was slow, and I often called in to see her and to keep her informed of what was going on at school. One day when I visited her she pointed to the tree outside the window and said, "You know, Jan, when the last leaf on that tree falls, I will go as well."

When her parents heard about this, they were obviously upset and her father hit upon the idea of painting an artificial leaf similar to the others. He did so, and fastened it to the tree while his daughter was asleep. He placed the artificial leaf in a position where she could clearly see it from her bed in front of the window. My little friend actually lived for quite a while after the real leaves had fallen. Although she continued to deteriorate, there was still some quality to her life and she still took pleasure in watching others getting on with their lives. Her parents made her as comfortable as possible, but eventually the day came when we had to say goodbye to her and she died peacefully.

This story could be seen as an allegory, symbolic of the possibilities of positive mind energy. This young girl had decided to outlive the last leaf on the tree and although she may have wondered about the unusual lifespan of that last remaining leaf, she did hang on.

It appears that more elderly people pass away in spring than in winter, even though the winter must be more taxing on their reserves than the gentler season of spring. The only logical explanation for this, to my mind, is that they are instinctively on their guard against the demands nature makes on their reserves in winter and are determined to see it out. Then spring comes and they feel they have achieved what they set out to do and can look forward to a time of relative peace. It is when they then let their guard down that nature takes its toll. When the older generation least suspects, nature will pounce and exact its demands.

People seem to need encouragement to transmute positive and negative thoughts into energy. The energy in our cells is influenced by our thoughts and mental vibrations. Kirlian photography can be used to show how cells are positively influenced and what the resulting energy aura is like. If you use this to check your thoughts, your judgements or anger, you will find that the energy aura alters according to your change of outlook. If you are in a joyous mood and feel like singing, or feel like helping someone whom you do not actually like, the energy in the cells will be greater as a result of such positive action. You will also find that the energy will increase as a result of a regular sleeping pattern or because of an improvement to your diet. Taking regular exercise and getting out into the fresh air will have similar effects, as oxygen is one of the best transmuters of energy, allowing more energy in the cell itself to be released.

We must become more conscious of the fact that thoughts and vibrations will bring harmony to mind, body and soul. I once heard an elderly professor tell his audience in a lecture that he always used to say good morning to his wife first thing in the morning, but that lately he had changed that habit of a lifetime to uttering a good morning to his body cells first and thanking them for keeping him alive and well. In today's demanding and stressful existence a positive attitude is more important than ever before, as our cellular system cannot be expected to resist such pressure without our conscious help and encouragement.

Positive thoughts are capable of curing ills, but only if we are sincere and truthful with ourselves. Our spoken words can belie what goes on in the mind and therefore sincerity must come from inside ourselves. In medicine it is not unknown for placebos to be prescribed. I have often pointed out to students the value of placebos, because they can work as neuro-transmitters, influencing action in order to produce innate energy. Balanced impulses and vibrations can lead to creative actions that in turn can result in ills being cured. No one can explain exactly how this works, but what we constantly find is that the intelligence that operates in every cell produces amazing results if the energy is directed correctly.

Some years ago I was approached by a lady who was totally and absolutely convinced that she was suffering from a fatal cancer. She told me that she had come to accept her illness because she had read articles on the subject and recognised the symptoms described as her own. Unfortunately, she had indoctrinated her mind into believing and accepting the fact that she had cancer and her energy had therefore been diminished. In that state of mind she could quite possibly have become prone to any illness. As I soon realised that she was a religious person, I pointed out to her Jesus' teachings on faith: "What things soever you desire, when you pray, believe that you receive them, and you shall have them" (Mark 11: v. 24).

I quoted this verse to her because a cancer cell, like any body cell, can be compared with a brain cell in that the cancer cell is also subject to positive thinking. Illness is the opposite of health, just as life is the opposite of death. Let us therefore gratefully accept the gift of life with a positive mind. If we use our energy positively, we can work miracles. We can then overcome illness and find peace.

God's gift of energy is in all of us, despite the fact that we often abuse it or fail to apply it. If we were to make use of this great gift of energy by programming the mind with a positive outlook, we would be able to help others as well as ourselves. The mind acting, is the mind thinking. The result of thinking is thought and the mind's action is the mind's thought. All thoughts, whether conscious or subconscious, are depressed, but many of them are expressed only in the organism of the thinker.

The mind and its energy is a wide subject. Consider the fact that the brain contains 14,000,000,000 cells and yet we cannot even define which part of it is responsible for our happiness, wisdom, intelligence, kindheartedness or common sense. We know sufficient, however, to steer us in the right direction and in this book you will find ways in which you can use your mind's energy positively, so as to produce an improvement in your well-being.

In 1775 an Austrian physician, Franz Anton Mesmer, introduced the word "biomagnetism" to the medical world. Through his experiments he showed that the mind can produce illness, i.e. psychosomatic illness. On the other hand he also proved that man can restore health by his own abilities and that hands are very often the most suitable energy conductor for this. In cases of psychosomatic problems a part of the temporal lobe in the visceral brain is often involved. This area of the brain links the negative emotions to the autonomic nervous system and the endocrine glands via the neopallum, the hypothalmus and the pituitary gland. The resulting intolerance on the part of the autonomic nervous system and the endocrine glands can lead to certain organic diseases that are often referred to as psychosomatic diseases, by releasing impulses that will inhibit the development of certain parts.

The prescription of medication will not always be successful in overcoming such conditions and relaxation exercises or autogenic training may be more beneficial. Let us not forget that the brain is the first organ of the body to respond; it acts as a receptor of our energy and how we positively influence our mind or brain depends entirely on our own actions.

To understand mind energy we first have to try to understand several underlying principles. In the first place the body has to work properly. All the organs have to function within each system. For this to happen there is need for the production of hormones and enzymes. This, in turn, requires vitamins, minerals and trace elements; these are transformed into enzymes to help digest the food we eat. When mind and body are in harmony and balanced, we will receive this wonderful energy which helps us to stay healthy, to perform our daily duties and to maintain an active and energetic life.

The human brain has both a positive and negative magnetic polar field. It is like a computer in some ways, but the brain of a human being or an animal is electro-magnetic. Moreover, the computer can only reproduce what is fed into it; it cannot think for itself. Let us have a positive mind as to what we feed into our computer, in order to obtain the means to live a positive and energetic life.

4

Energy in the Endocrine

I DOUBT IF ever before in the history of the existence of mankind the endocrine system has been under more severe strain than at present. Not even specialist endocrinologists will claim to fully understand this system. All we know is that it is closely linked to man's emotions and inner feelings. The endocrines are not only subject to attack by adverse atmospheric influences, but also, one could say, by the spirits of our time.

Let us consider the seven small glands that make up the endocrine system and the worthwhile functions they perform. Then we will be able to appreciate the need for further in-depth studies of these glands. A homoeopathic or naturopathic practitioner will never separate the physical actions of the endocrine glands from their spiritual actions. And we are well aware that if one of these glands is out of harmony, all seven glands will suffer, because this disturbs the balance of the whole endocrine system.

One great influence on maintaining a good harmony and balance in body energies is atmospheric or innate energy. We often see patients who are clinically depressed because of hormonal problems caused by a disharmony somewhere between these seven glands. Even though they may appear to be of insignificant size, each gland has an extremely important function and should always be regarded as an ally within the human body.

Let us consider what controls these seven glands and what influences them. The science of endocrinology embraces all the internal secretions of these ductless glands. These secretions are very potent and are essential for all living organisms. The nutrition we obtain from our food is regulated by these glands, so is the degree of vitality that influences the condition of our skin, the colour of our hair, and the strength of our muscles. The endocrines are also instrumental in the functions of the liver, stomach and intestines and help to determine the entire electrical potential in the human body.

Although our knowledge of the medical or physical aspects of the pineal gland is far from complete, we know that this little gland, which often has metaphysical associations, secretes fluids that are decisive in the growth and development of sexual organs. As the pineal gland is subject to atmospheric influences, it is frequently called "the third eye". Any imbalance in energy is often the result of the pineal gland not functioning to its maximum capacity. Sometimes the pineal gland is also referred to as "the spirit of love", because it is influenced by emotions and, negatively, by lack of regard.

The pituitary gland is said to be the key to the chemistry of the whole of the body. The pituitary hormones chemically affect the cell membranes. Therefore the chemical reactions do not work properly when the pituitary gland is in any way impaired or prevented from doing its correct job. This gland is situated at the nasal suture, the place where the nose meets the forehead. An imbalance in this gland can affect the normal growth pattern of children, while in adults it can cause impotence in men or irregular menstruation in women. The severity of diabetes can also be determined by the pituitary gland.

In order to function properly the pituitary gland needs a good intake of vegetable protein, which is very important for the production of hormones and also for the different enzymes in the body. This gland is often referred to as the "master gland" or "conductor of the endocrine orchestra" and it releases hormones to either promote or inhibit the release of other endocrine hormones. Indirectly, it controls such basic processes as rate of growth, metabolic rate, water and electrolyte balance, kidney filtration, ovulation and lactation. It responds to hormones released by the region of the brain known as the hypothalmus, and is a physical link between the nervous and the endocrine system.

Next we have the thyroid gland, which is situated at the front of the trachea. This gland also influences the metabolic processes, which ultimately affect the whole nervous system. Body energy is extremely dependent on a well-functioning thyroid gland and will be affected if there are problems in this respect. The thyroid is a glandular link between the brain and the reproductive organs and it is certain that it can be triggered or inhibited by emotional disturbances, directly influencing circulation, respiration and tissue growth and repair. Over-production of thyroxine from the thyroid gland will lead to problems in these processes and, equally, so will under-production. We often see how individuals are emotionally affected when a thyroid defect appears. Thus it becomes apparent why this gland is also known as "the spirit of life".

The pancreas is best described by likening it to a small bunch of grapes situated across the posterior wall of the abdomen. This gland secretes pancreatic fluid, which regulates the glucose contents of the body tissues that rely on this fluid. Digestive enzymes are secreted into the small intestine, which produces hormones for release into the blood. The digestive enzymes are crucial, because the incorrect breakdown of ingested fats, proteins and sugars can lead to digestive complaints such as diabetes or hypoglycaemia.

The thymus gland is often underrated, as it is generally believed that its level of productivity decreases after puberty, eventually falling to about 10 per cent of its original level by the age of forty. It is, however, amiss to claim that this gland is of no importance, because it fully deserves the name "gland of purification and immunity", by which it is also known. Especially when we consider the pollution of air and water prevalent today, we come to realise that the role played by this gland is possibly more important than ever before. It cannot possibly be true that this gland loses its usefulness and this fact becomes quite clear when we look at a patient with the muscular complaint myasthenia gravis.

One of my patients who suffered from this condition was determined to get this problem sorted out quickly and effectively and therefore agreed to have his thymus gland surgically removed. Certainly the myasthenia gravis condition disappeared, but had I not seen it for myself, I doubt if I would have believed the change of character and personality this person underwent. Moreover, this was not the only change that he experienced; it was equally clear that his immunity had been badly impaired as a result of this operation and therefore other problems quickly reared their head. Again I will stress that if one of these glands is affected, the whole endocrine system will become imbalanced and this alone should be sufficient reason to avoid surgery on any of these seven glands, except where there seems to be no other solution.

Then there are the adrenals — small, yellowish triangular bodies — situated one above each of the kidneys. The functions of the adrenals are closely related to the autonomic nervous system and the adrenal secretion regulates the blood pressure. When we realise that the adrenals produce fifty different natural steroid hormones, we cannot fail to recognise the importance of these glands. Some of these hormones are involved in the conversion of dietary protein and fat into glucose, while others suppress inflammation and promote healing. The blood/iron balance in the kidneys is also regulated by adrenal hormones. Any adverse influence on the adrenal secretion can affect the oxydisation process that regulates the circulatory system. The principal hormone produced, called adrenaline, will be ready to respond to any emergency. Good nutrition, exercise and water are needed for the adrenals to function correctly.

Last, but not least, we come to the gonad glands — the male and female sexual endocrine glands — which are essential for the reproduction of the species. The gonads produce internal secretions that are distributed by the blood in order to stimulate and revitalise all other glands and organs in the body, and therefore they also create a certain amount of external secretion. To my thinking the gonad glands have a role to play in present-day problems such as AIDS. I therefore believe that in the case of AIDS patients treatment with natural remedies which influence the gonads may produce significant benefits.

These seven very important endocrine glands are often treated with a lack of respect, and we ought to remember that they are very sensitive from both a mental and physical viewpoint. It is not sufficient to treat them correctly with pure food, water and air, they also respond to exercise, prayer and meditation. Let us not overlook the fact that they are very closely linked to the seven *shakras*, or the seven sources of spiritual energy — the description used in the Far East for energy centres in the body whose counterparts are present in the physical body of the glandular and nervous system.

The locations of these seven sources of spiritual energy are as follows:

Pituitary gland — the ground *shakra*
Pineal gland — the "third eye" or the forehead *shakra*
Thyroid — the neck *shakra*
Thymus — the heart *shakra*
Pancreas — the sun *shakra*
Adrenals — the sacral *shakra*
Gonads — the root *shakra*

These descriptive Far Eastern names for the seven *shakras* indicate the need for physical care as well as spiritual exercise, if we are to help these energy centres to awaken and activate their healing powers, which are often dormant, in order to attain full harmony between mind, body and spirit. Physical and mental exercise serves to strengthen all the vital functions and to maintain good health and because it is conducive to a good energy flow, there will be no place for illness or disease.

In addition to the seven endocrine glands there are five other energy centres in the human body of equal importance. If there is a disturbance anywhere in these energy channels an imbalance could result that may cause an energy blockage. In these circumstances acupuncture treatment can often restore the balance in these energies. It is also sometimes possible to reactivate them using simple vibrations. The crown of these energies lies in an area of the pituitary gland, which is considerably influenced by cosmic energy. In the Far East I have also heard the pituitary gland referred to as the "energy centre of faith" and the gonads described as the "energy centre of life", or sometimes the "new earth".

To condense briefly what I intended to say in this chapter, the endocrine system has a great need for physical, mental and spiritual balance and any energy disturbances can lead to further problems that could often have been avoided. Lack of due care or consideration in maintaining this balance can cause, for example, hardening of the arteries, rheumatism, arthritis, brain degeneration, ossification, impaired hearing or sight, anaemia, forgetfulness or constipation. This fact underlines how important it is that these glands are constantly nurtured and stimulated. This can be done, for example, by cranial osteopathy, endocrine foot reflexology or acupuncture. If these therapies are not sufficiently effective, I also occasionally prescribe glandular extracts for patients who are in need.

You may be surprised to learn that breathing exercises can also help to regain a balance in the endocrine system.

It may be helpful to look at Chapter 8 on energy of the feet, which describes simple methods for generally improving the body energy balance. A diagram showing the endocrine reflexes in the feet is also given on page 122.

The secret of maintaining a balance in the endocrine system is to bring into harmony the qualities of body energy and it is true that by conscientious application of the simple techniques mentioned in this book relief can be gained from tension and exhaustion. Many a time I have seen patients who had been deeply depressed and even suicidal regain mental stability with the help of such simple methods or exercises. Heeding advice concerning positive thinking can lead to a better quality of life. In this connection, too, not only is our daily intake of food and drink important, but it should also be remembered that atmospheric influences need to be considered.

I recently treated a patient about whom I was greatly concerned because of the rate at which he was depleting his immune system. He spoke to me about the conditions he worked under and a few things then became clear to me. His place of work was lit by fluorescent lights and he was surrounded by word processors and computers. The general pressure this amounted to was clearly taking its toll. This brings to mind the coincidence of the number seven. Is it really coincidental that apart from the endocrine system having seven glands, the solar spectrum also has seven colours, that there are seven layers of light receptors in the retina of the eye and that there are seven basic scale steps in a musical octave.

The condition of this patient proved yet again how important environmental and atmospheric conditions are to the immune system and to that end a well-functioning endocrine system is vital. In the next chapter we will see how excellent a mirror the eyes are of the energy present in the endocrines.

5

Energy in the Eyes

FROM STUDYING THE endocrine system we have come to realise that the eyes play an important part in the general harmony of the body and ultimately act like mirrors of what is happening inside. Often, signs of an imbalance or disharmony in the body can be detected in the eyes. It is therefore even more worrying that the modern technology of visual display units can have such a detrimental influence on the eyes, as well as weakening the endocrine system generally. Working continuously in areas lit by fluorescent lights also serves to diminish the effective functioning of the endocrine system and, ultimately, that person's immunity.

A good way of showing that the above is true is to take a Kirlian photograph of someone who has just come in from being in the daylight after having been there for some time. Then let him work for an hour or longer under fluorescent lights before taking another photograph. While the first photograph will most likely depict a reasonably good energy aura, you will find that the same aura will undoubtedly be impaired on the second photograph. The same effect becomes apparent after someone has been watching television for some time, or has been working at a word processor, peering at the monitor screen.

Our eyes are very delicate and sensitive and because my parents and immediate family do not possess very good eyesight, I am only too aware of the precious gift of sight. I have treated people who were almost blind, some with more success than others. But if we ever wonder what it would be like not to be able to see, imagine how terrible it would be if all the colour and variety of forms that fill the world around us were absent. Even the senses of touch and smell become secondary when we consider their dependence on an initial impression of sight.

Vision depends on several factors — three to be precise. Firstly, light is required; secondly the brain, nerves and eyes must be able to function and thirdly, what the eyes are able to record, and how this is done, depends on the interests of the individual.

The retina consists of nerve tissue, which in a developing unborn baby is actually part of the brain itself. You may be surprised to learn that there are 137 million sight-receiving cells located in the retina, which connect with about one million "telephone lines" as it were, which in turn connect with the sight centre of the brain. Sight is such a wonderful creation and most of the time we just take it for granted! Our ignorance becomes obvious when we see certain people who are losing their sight still glued to the television screen for hours on end. This ignorance also displays itself in our food intake. Vulnerable persons must make extra sure that their food contains an ample supply of vitamin A, which is extremely important for our eyesight.

The eyes themselves have a marvellous power of accommodation, which enables them to do their wonderful work. Not only do they enable us to see, but they also give the spectator or outsider a chance to see what is happening inside us. The eyes are often called "the mirror of the soul" — and this is not just a poetic phrase.

The eyes provide us with a finely tuned analysis of our biochemistry and of emotional and circumstantial factors which are hard to determine in any other way. Iridology is the science of analysing the delicate structure of the iris of the eye and any disturbance in energy will be picked up by a good iridologist. In this way he will find out if any aspect of the body is out of harmony. Under the magnification of a biomicroscope the iris reveals itself as a world of minute details. It is a complete map that represents a communication system capable of handling an amazing quantity of information. The iris is an extension of the brain, and is prolifically endowed with hundreds and thousands of nerve endings, microscopic blood vessels and other tissue.

Each iris is connected to every organ and tissue of the body via the brain and the nervous system. The nerve fibres receive their impulses by way of convection from the optic nerve, optic thalamus and spinal cord. They are formed embriologically from mesoderm and neuro-ectoderm tissue and both the sympathetic and para-sympathetic nervous system are represented in the iris. In this way, nature has provided us with a miniature television screen showing the most remote parts of the body, which normally cannot be seen by conventional diagnostic methods using nerve reflex responses.

Isn't it wonderful to think that through the body's natural X-ray equipment, i.e. the eyes, we can perceive, intelligently and accurately, how the life force moves and operates, enabling us to diagnose accordingly. Most people, however, have no idea that every abnormality in the physical body and every perversity in the mental sphere is clearly impressed upon the iris.

We first learned about this in 1881, when the Hungarian physician Ignaz von Pēczēly wrote a paper on this subject. At the age of eleven, while playing in his family's garden, he captured an owl. In the struggle that ensued the bird sustained a broken leg. After the owl had been subdued, the observant boy noticed a white cloud in the lower part of the bird's iris on the same side of its body as the injured leg. When the leg had healed and he looked into the bird's iris again, he noticed that a black speck circumscribed by white lines had replaced the former cloud-like sign. Years later, when Pēczēly was a practising physician, he was called up to treat a man who had a fractured leg. When he examined the man, he was once more confronted with the curious spot in the patient's iris, similar to the one he had observed in the owl. From then on he continued his investigations and discovered various definite areas in the iris that corresponded with the different parts of the body. Meanwhile, unbeknown to him, a Swede, a Frenchman and a Dane were also studying the same subject and they, too, were reaching the same conclusions as Pēczēly.

It is a good thirty years now since a Dutch doctor, Dr N. Bos, introduced me to iridology in our clinic in the Netherlands. I would not like to think how I would ever have coped without my subsequent knowledge and continued study of iridology. That study never ends and I still find iridology to be of tremendous help in reaching a diagnosis for certain health problems with my patients.

Iridology has been subject to much criticism. Yet how would we be able to determine a person's characteristics if we could not see that person? In the same way, if we did not have a mirror of body and soul we would not be able to look deeper into that person. In China I have also learned how to conduct facial diagnosis, with the help of which I can easily discover where energy in the human body might be disturbed, but this differs from the science of iridology in that the latter is based on the eyes only.

The correlation of circumstances and expression is a certainty. An experienced doctor can generally see from the condition of the skin or other external symptoms what is happening inside his patient and this is also the case with iridology. Even a thousand years before Christ the Chaldeans were aware of, and practised, eye diagnostics and in ancient astrological books one is able to read about how it was applied in those days. If the body is healthy and has enough energy for its requirements, then the iris will show a nice even structure. If there is a light-dark mark, or a discoloration or cloud, then the iridologist will take great care to discover what may be wrong and where.

In my work as an acupuncturist I can actually see changes taking place when I position needles on certain energy points; immediately a difference is noticeable in the iris. When the energy level is diminished during periods of nervous anxiety or depression, the iris will portray what is occurring both in physical terms and mentally.

The Evangelist Luke, who was a trained and practising physician, wrote:

> The light of the body is the eye: therefore when thine eye is single thy whole body also is full of light; but when thine eye is evil, the body also is full of darkness. (Luke 11: v. 34).

These words are a clear indication that even in those days it was known that the eyes portrayed signs of a person's physical and mental well-being. As far as the endocrine system is concerned, the eyes certainly are the mirror of body and soul.

In some of my earlier books I have mentioned my work with prisoners who serve a life sentence. In interviews with them I can obtain a fairly accurate impression of their mental and physical condition by studying their faces and in particular their eyes, which often signal an imbalance between mind and body.

In this book, however, it is my intention to concentrate on energy. The nervous system is the medium that transmits signals and messages to the iris. When the fibres of the iris are close together, the person has a strong energy picture. When, however, those fibres are loosely woven, broken or distorted, then energy and vitality are lacking and the person is unable to withstand disease, or attacks from viruses or infections.

Colour therapy often proves beneficial under such circumstances. Vision will improve in response to being exposed to the different colours of light radiation for a certain period. The light vibrationary energy mostly found in the colour blue will have a sedative effect; the colour red, on the other hand, stimulates and the colour green helps to relieve congestion.

Colour therapy is only part of the treatment that can be applied to the eyes. So much more can be done in this field. Not only do we receive diagnostic messages from the eyes, but often they offer us the scope to re-energise the person concerned, or to help them obtain relief from certain conditions. Unimpaired vision is, of course, most important and for this, colour therapy offers great energising possibilities. When using colour treatment for healing purposes it deals with the finest vibrations in nature which are so much more beneficial to the body than the irritation caused by drugs or chemicals.

Radiation from sunlight is absorbed by the nervous system and distributed by the bloodstream to the various parts of the body. If a weak energy is stimulated by red colours, Kirlian photography will show the improvement in the aura obtained after the colour treatment. I have used this technique to prove the efficacy of this treatment to sceptics and have been able to point out the original energy disturbances and the resulting reduction in the imbalance after the treatment.

The laws of nature are basically very simple. As long as we appreciate the healing powers of nature, the evidence will speak for itself after having treated patients physically, mentally or emotionally. When we see a rainbow in the sky we are reminded of great promise. The same is true of the colours used in colour therapy.

Energy for the eyes — what better advice can I give you than to aim to protect your eyes from the stress and strain of modern life. Is this still possible? Let us every now and then venture to keep away from electric light, television screens and visual display units, and really give our eyes the chance to rest. This measure is especially advisable for people who suffer from eye strain or a burning sensation in the eyes. If we give the eyes a rest from all that is artificial, not only will the eyes benefit, but the whole body.

Nature has supplied us with a number of remedies that provide us with some extra help. The herb eyebright, as the name indicates, or marigold tea, or Dr Vogel's Galeopsis will all help to restore the essential energy balance in the eyes. Careful palpation of the eyeballs through the upper lids will help to relieve tension. Apply a pumping motion and gradually increase the downward pressure for the count of five or ten. Then quickly release and repeat. This will accomplish some useful drainage of the eyeball. Tapping your finger over the eyeball will also prove helpful. A good manipulation for the eyes, when the energy level is down, is the following, more general, technique. Carefully place a finger of the left hand on each eye, with the lids closed. Grasp the lids with the right hand and very gently make them vibrate. This is a most energising and relaxing treatment for the eyes, and can be done without any danger whatsoever.

Scientists and technicians from all over the world have contributed to the knowledge of vision and are continuing with their work to help us to learn about the complex processes of vision, which is so important for a balanced harmony in mind and body. The importance of vision is aptly expressed in yet another biblical saying:

> Where there is no vision, the people perish
> (Proverbs 29: v. 18).

6

Energy in the Hands

IS OUR HEALTH in our own hands? I have often drawn attention, in my lectures and in my books, to the tremendous energy and power we possess in our own hands. However, we need to learn how to use our hands to channel this energy and where to apply pressure when energy is disturbed. For generations people have known that they were able to influence the balance of their energies by means of pressure and massage using their hands. Unfortunately, in modern times these faculties have fallen into disuse. We have become too "civilised". The basic facts, however, have not changed. We once had this gift and, fortunately, some people have managed to retain it.

Our hands can be used for many different purposes. As humans, from infancy we use our hands instinctively when expressing our thoughts or purposes. The hands, therefore, are a tool on which the mind depends for expressive action. For some people their hands have actually become their only means of communication. Many profoundly deaf people rely totally on their hands as a means of expressing themselves.

NATURE'S GIFT

In this chapter I would like to concentrate on our ability to use our hands to help people who suffer, by easing their pain. Our hands can be used to ease a large variety of health problems, largely by placing them in the right places at the right times.

Some time ago I visited some primitive tribes and was amazed yet again to see how they had the ability to use their hands in such a way that they could ease pain and quickly solve a variety of health problems. They showed me how to restore the energy balance in seconds, but I could not begin to copy their technique. I would certainly need a lot more time if I intended to treat my patients with similar methods. It was wonderful to watch them completely solve a patient's complaints merely by placing a thumb on the corresponding energy point. I have learned an enormous amount from these people on the subject of rebalancing energy in the body and using energy to our best advantage. I have watched them treat even a slipped disc without any manipulation and greatly admire their inborn abilities.

Let me make it clear that this treatment method bears no relation at all to the so-called "laying on of hands" or faith healing, in any form. The method I describe involves a scientific knowledge of the energy within, which can be balanced as long as we know where to find the appropriate energy points. The laws of nature are simple, as I have said before, and healing too can be simple. We often tend to over-complicate the procedure and it is then that we can learn a valuable lesson from those so-called "primitives". They have remained in close touch with nature, whereas we seem to have moved further and further away.

In ancient civilisations, it appears, it was already known the right hand has a positive power compared to a negative power in the left hand. This fact has since been confirmed. Whether one is male or female has no bearing on this, nor does the fact that one is left-handed or right-handed. All that is important is that the hands are used at the right times in the right places. The palm of the right hand has a positive energy and the left hand conducts negative energy and when the correct balance is found, great benefits can be achieved.

The energy in one's hands is like a vital force that circulates through the body on specific pathways. It is stimulated to heal or to prevent functional imbalance and it depends on the south pole energy — in the right hand — which will strengthen the biological systems and effect an increase in overall strength. The right hand should never be used on infections, as it carries a positive charge. The left hand affords relief from pain and has the ability to arrest or slow down an infection, reducing nerve pains, swellings and strengthening weak muscles.

I have found that one very good exercise to energise oneself is to place the right hand over the forehead and the left hand over the neck exactly over the occipit. On holding this for a little while one will experience a renewed energy flow. The same thing happens when we place the right hand on the stomach under the navel and cover this with the left hand. This is the way to energise Hara — the seat of energy — and almost within seconds one feels recharged. The effect is almost comparable to when one's car battery is recharged after it has been running low. The positive pole is connected to the positive pole of electricity and the negative pole to the negative electric charge and the battery will be recharged. By using the hands as described, one can achieve similar effects for the body in order to relieve a stressed area or regain additional energy.

The ancient Chinese already knew that the abdominal area could be stimulated to produce reflexes that might help them. They knew that this was particularly so for the area around the navel and used this knowledge to their advantage. The left hand is placed on the painful zone and the right hand on the spinal area immediately behind it. In this way many problems can be relieved, such as those affecting the heart, gallbladder, stomach, kidneys, lungs, spleen, liver, small intestine, colon and bladder. These parts of the body are all centred around the navel and this bears out the validity of the navel sometimes being called the "abdominal brain", as it is through this area that energy intake occurs.

It is interesting that healing by placing the hands in certain positions has been practised for centuries. It is with gratitude to my dear friend Dr (Ac.) Leonard J. Allan DO, that I am now able to list some of the specific positions he has gathered over the years from various sources.

For hundreds of years special hand positions have been used as part of rituals or meditation, particularly in religious activities. In the Christian tradition there is the position of the hands held together in devotion. In the Buddhist tradition there are the positions of the "quiet hands", characteristic of so many statues of Buddha. An observation of people in many cultures, or of paintings and pictures of them, yields a number of different hand positions. In many cases these positions are assumed unconsciously by the individual merely because the position is comfortable. Nevertheless, the assumed position is often appropriate to the physical, emotional or mental attitude or motivation of the individual.

In the last few years a subjective investigation of the nervous system within the context of meditation has shed considerable light on the significance of these hand positions and has led to the discovery of a host of others of even greater importance for the student of self-improvement. It has been learned that there are a number of "connection points" in the nervous system which, when brought into proximity by the appropriate body position, set up nerve circuits which induce specific mind-body functions. In combination, a great number of mind-body functions can be induced, some of which can be of great benefit to the individual, since they in turn augment various forms of healing when that term is used in its broadest sense to include the physical, emotional, mental and spiritual aspects of existence.

Hand positions

The hand positions described below will help the individual

to achieve specific rebalancing and will also promote a general improvement in mind-body balance. Depending on the individual, the effectiveness of some positions may diminish after repeated use, whereas others will be found beneficial even after they have been used many times.

The hand positions illustrated are not always symmetrical, i.e. one hand may be held in a different manner to the other one. Thus, when trying a particular position, one may feel more comfortable with left and right hands reversed as compared to the position as illustrated. In such a case, the more comfortable position should always be used. There is often a difference between the preference of men and women in this respect, as a result of their opposite polarities from left to right.

The vast majority of the hand positions will not draw undue attention to the user and certain ones will be of great benefit when used in the presence of others, particularly in the presence of persons who are using energy to the detriment of others around them.

Some of the positions, however, will provide the most benefit in rebalancing or meditation when practised while alone and a number of these will be beneficial even when practised while the user is sleeping. The use of a stocking or other device may be required to hold the hands in the desired position, thus dispensing with the need for the conscious mind to concentrate on holding the position.

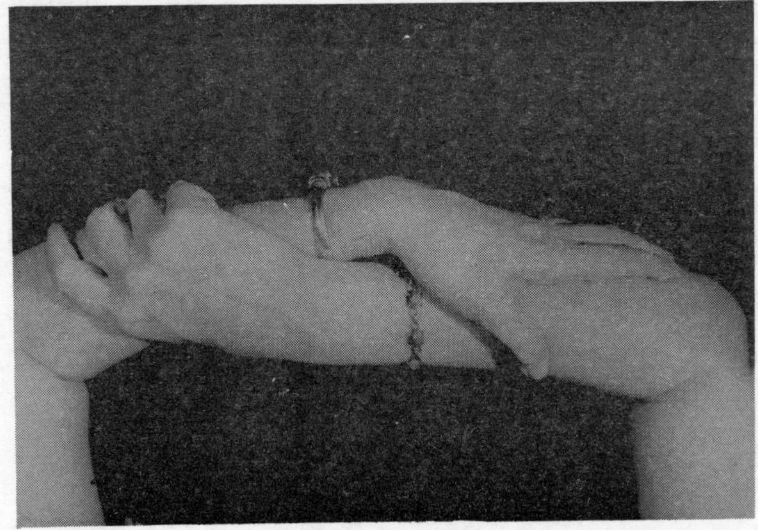

Own true self (1)

This position is used to bring the sense of action to rest. It is useful for isolating oneself in the presence of moderate energy. Each forearm is grasped by the opposite hand. The ankles may also be crossed at the same time.

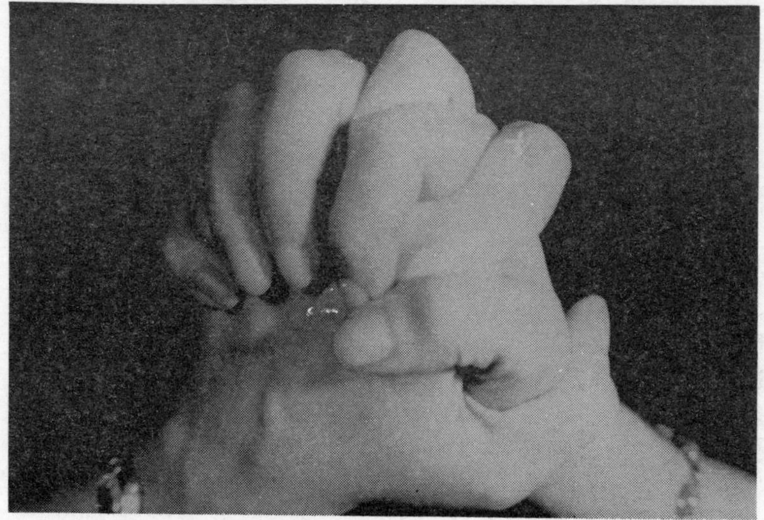

Own true self (2)

This is used to induce quiet perception. (The hands are clasped, with the fingers and thumbs externally intertwined.)

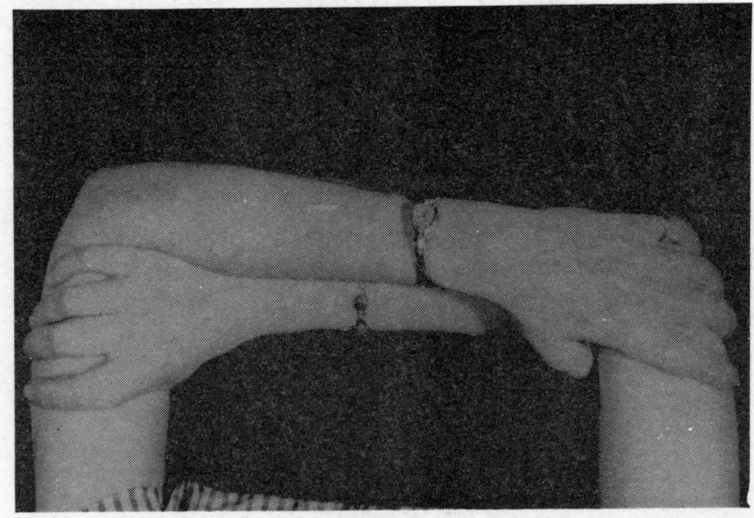

Own true self (3)

Use this position to isolate oneself in the presence of heavy and disturbing energy. (The upper arm is grasped by the opposite hand.)

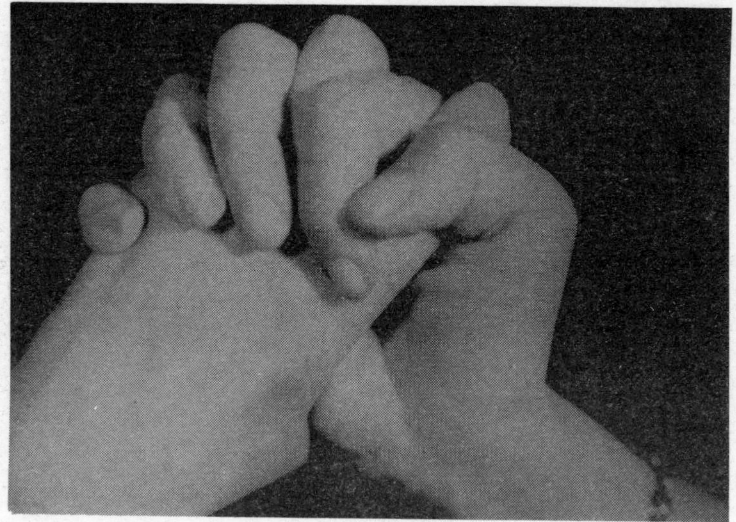

Own true self (4)

This position is used to balance our valencies. (The fingers and thumbs are externally intertwined, with the free thumb placed under the wrist of the other hand.)

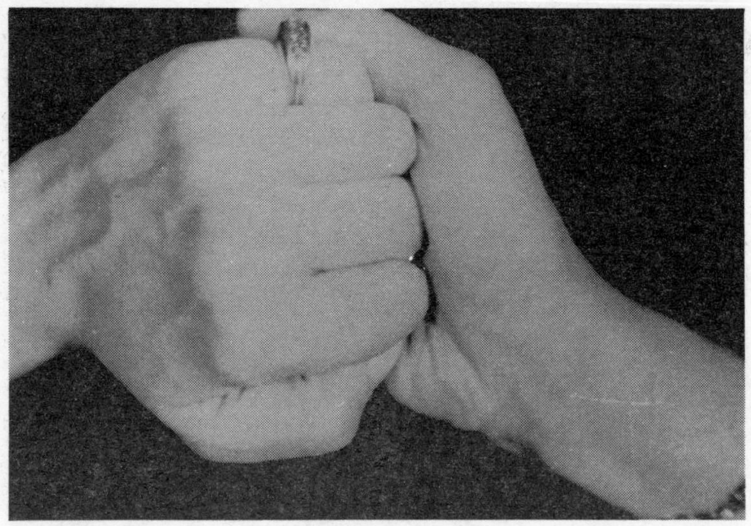

Keying things out

This position helps to calm a person down. It also has a neutralising effect on various part of the body, such as the stomach and eyes. (The fingers of each hand are hooked and firmly engage each other. Each thumb lies along the little finger of the opposite hand.)

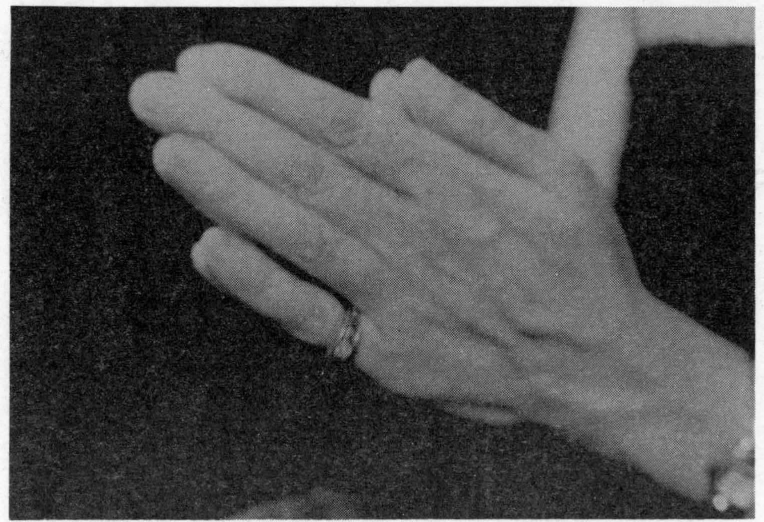

Devotion

(The hands are stretched flat and placed together as in the traditional position for prayer.)

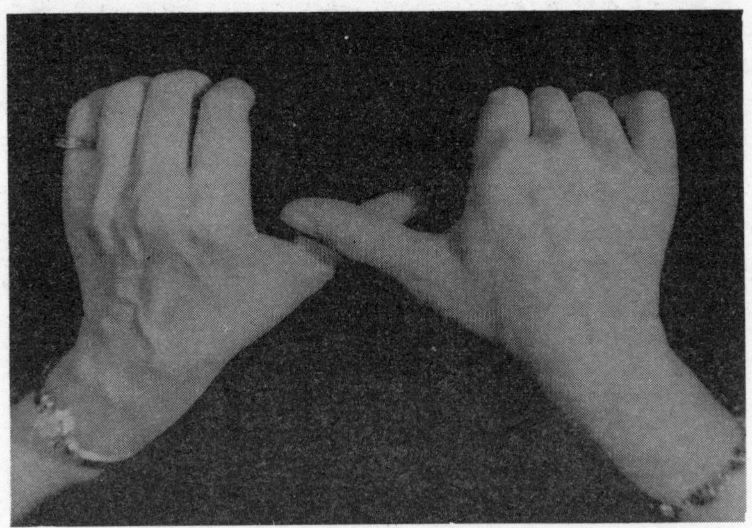

Step 1

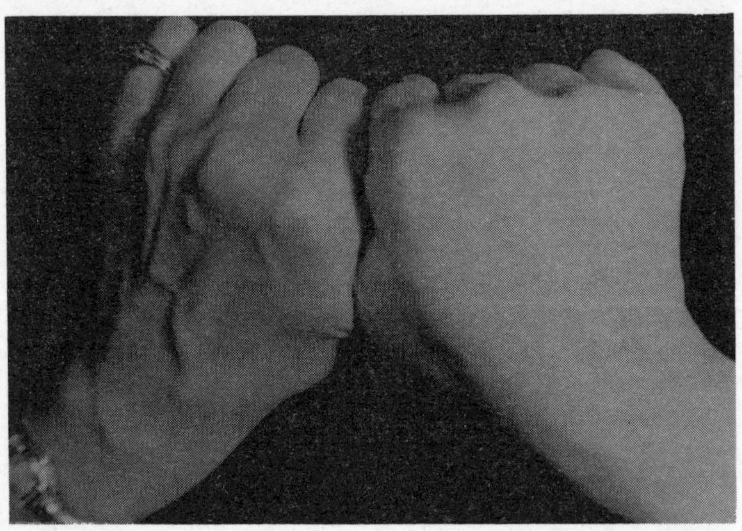

Step 2

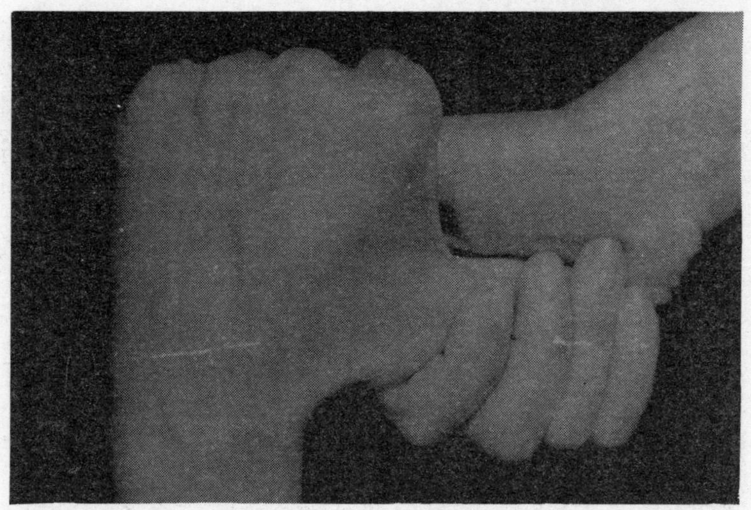

Getting in the positive

Use this position to correct negative attitudes. (This is the same position as the previous one, except that the hands are rotated so that one wrist is up and the other wrist is down.)

Sending attending energies in point

This position is used to send attending energies automatically to where they are needed at any point in the body. It can be used for breaking up congestions. (The thumb of each hand is grasped between the fingers and palm of the opposite hand. The position is easily entered by first crossing the thumbs (*Step 1*) and sliding the hands together before closing the fingers (*Step 2*).)

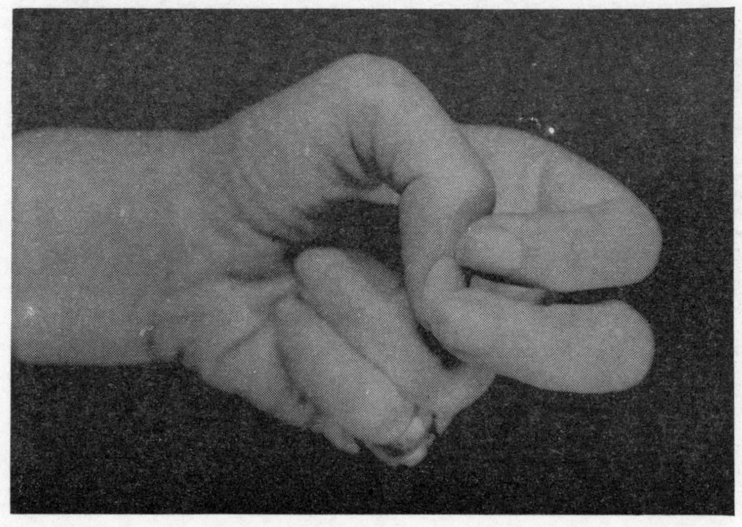

Activating without energy

This position helps to keep the mind alert in the absence of energy and is used when the hands cannot be brought together. (The fourth and little fingers are held against the palm and the tips of the forefinger and middle finger are placed on the first digit of the thumb.)

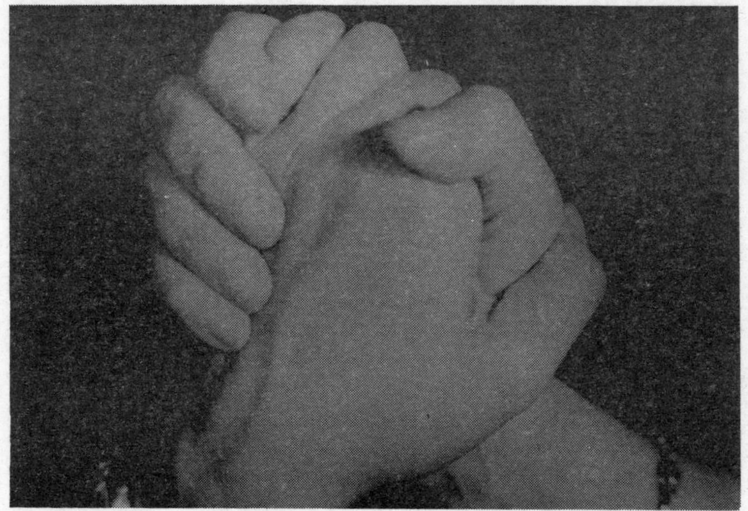

Foreground awareness

This position promotes the inner self and also serves to de-energise. (With the fingers held together, the palms are placed to face each other at right angles and then the fingers and thumbs are wrapped around the opposite hand.)

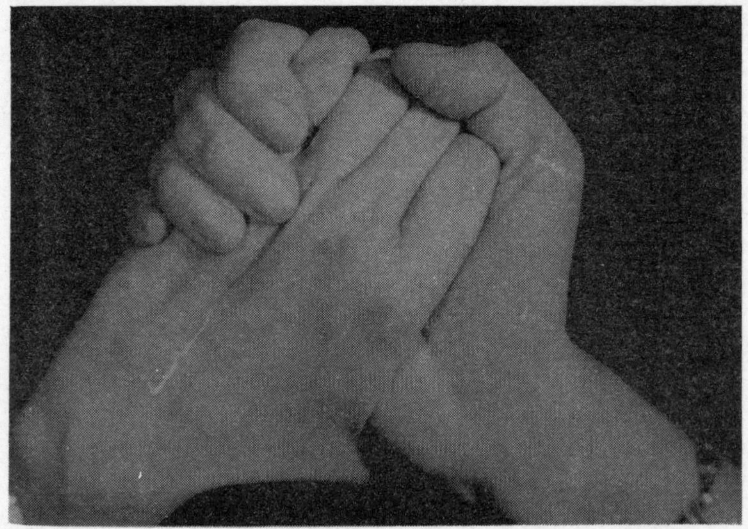

Background awareness

This is used to pull oneself together and protect one from energy domination by another person. This is the same as the previous clasp, except that the free thumb is placed behind the opposite wrist.)

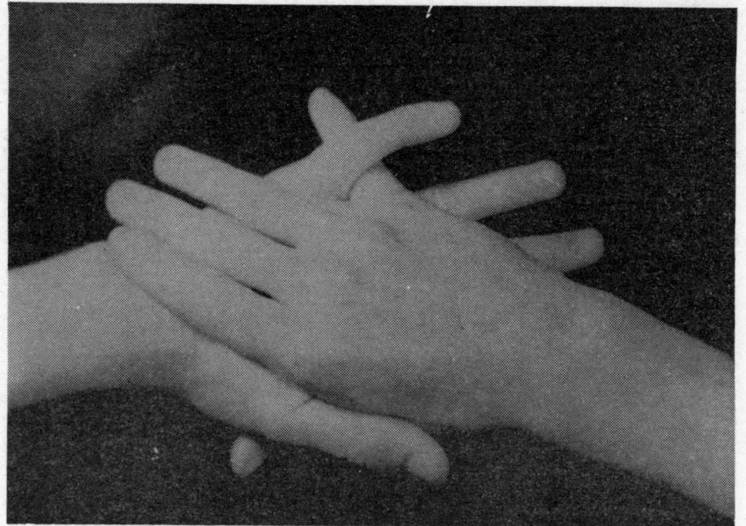

Without willpower

This position helps one to release the emotions that have been withheld. (The palm of one hand is placed on the back of the other hand. The thumbs and little fingers are interlocked.)

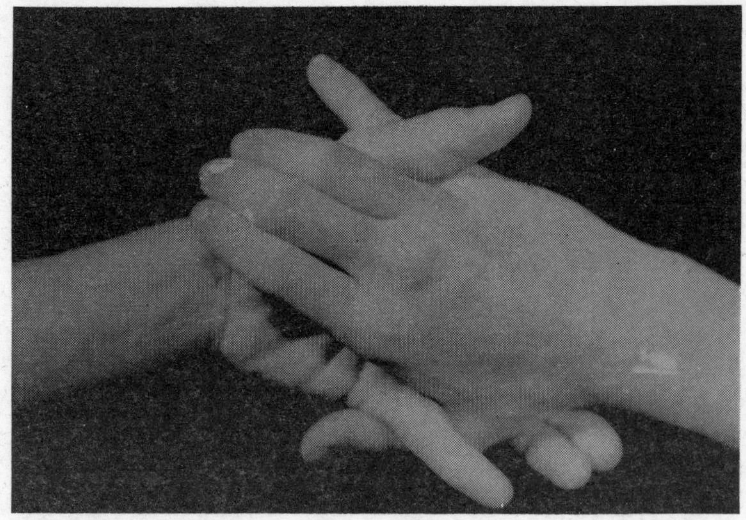

As of now

This position has an immediate impact on the senses and aids rebalancing. (The hands are held flat and placed palm to palm. The thumb of each hand is interlocked with the little finger of the opposite hand.)

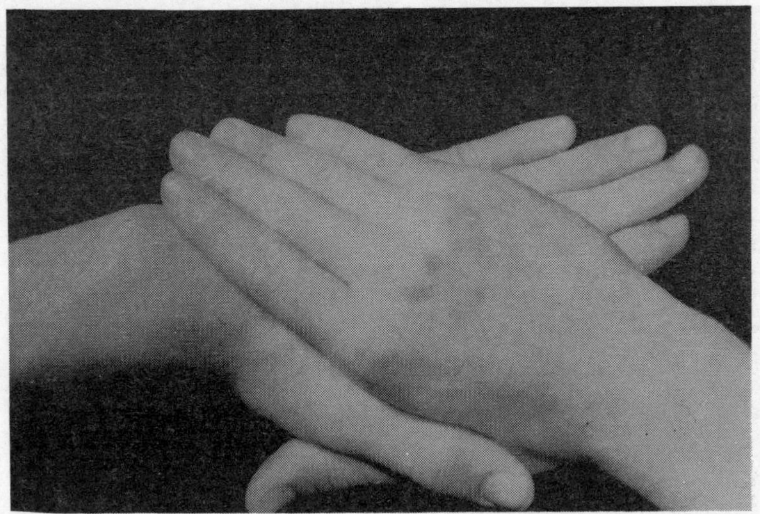

Neutralising

This position promotes a calm mind and aids in meditation. It also neutralises unbalanced body conditions when the hands are held in this way and placed over a deficient body part such as tense stomach. (One hand is held flat and placed on the back of the other and the thumbs are interlocked.)

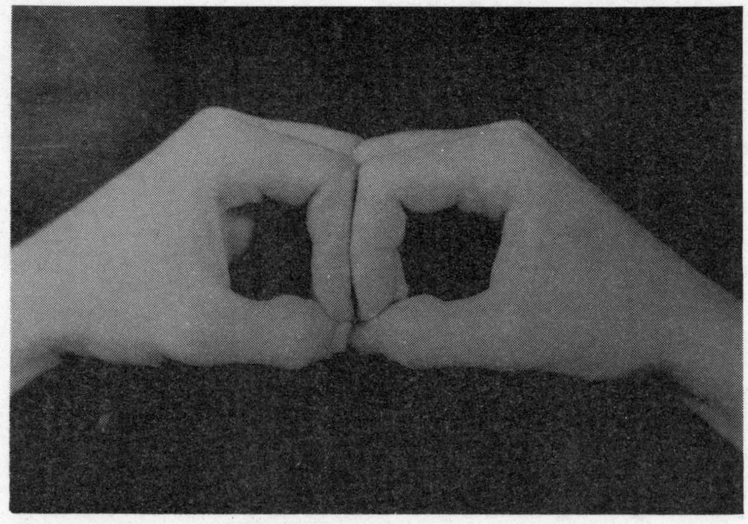

Quiet hands (1)

This position is used to quieten the forebrain. (The fingertips are placed in line and bent over to make a circle, with each thumb tip touching the tip of the forefinger. The backs of the knuckles of all the fingers are brought together.)

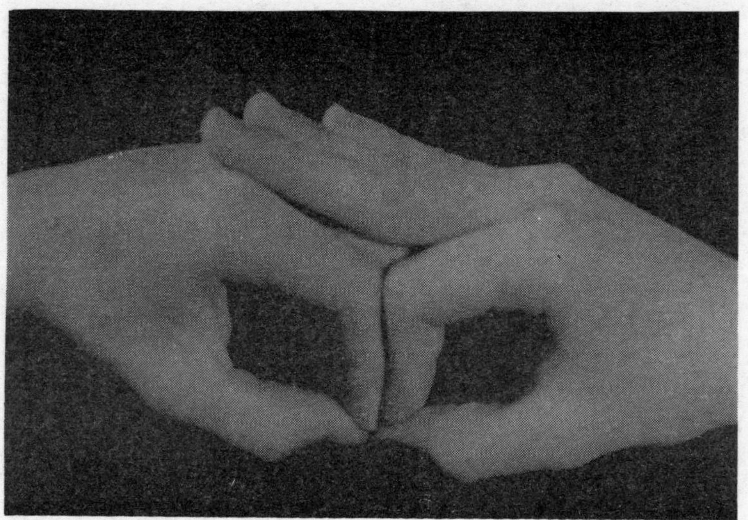

Quiet hands (2)

This quietens the midbrain. (A circle is made with each thumb and forefinger, with the three remaining fingers of each hand remaining extended and together. The extended fingers of one hand are placed on top of those of the other hand.)

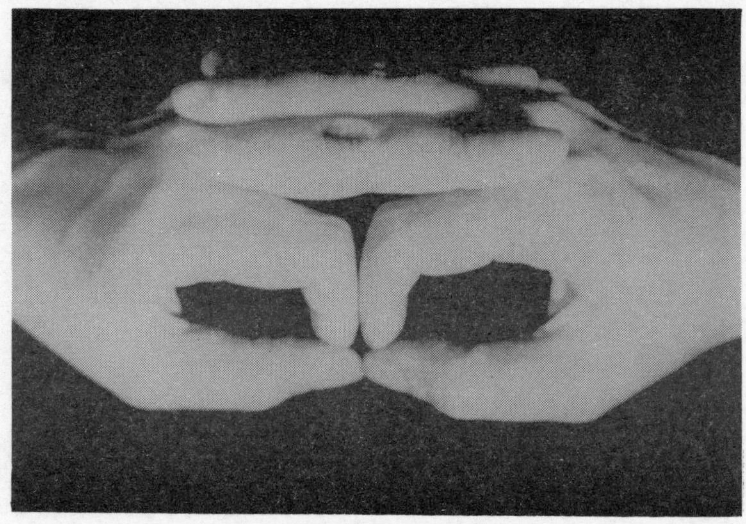

Quiet hands (3)

This quietens the hindbrain. (This is the same as the previous position, except that the extended fingers are externally intertwined, or interlaced.)

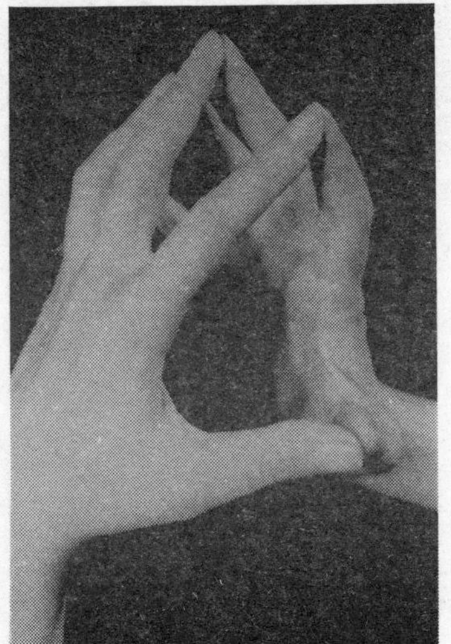
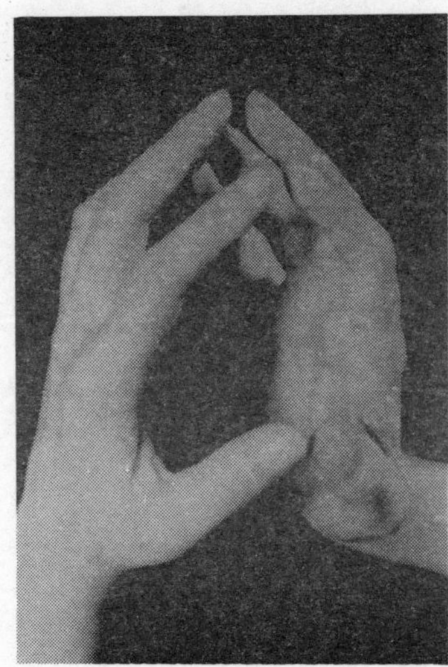

Talking without energy

This position improves the flow of energy from one person to another. It also keeps the mind on business rather than personalities. (With the fingers spread apart, a cup is made out of each hand. The corresponding fingertips are brought together and then separated again by about half an inch. Do this once every 1-2 seconds, or even less often if that seems more comfortable.)

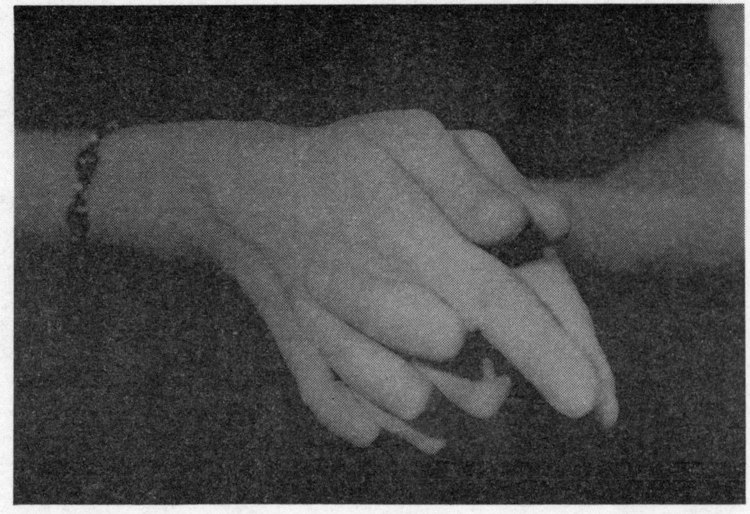

Rebalancing forehead blocks

(The little fingers, fourth fingers and middle fingers are intertwined externally. The thumbs and forefingers are held alongside each other.)

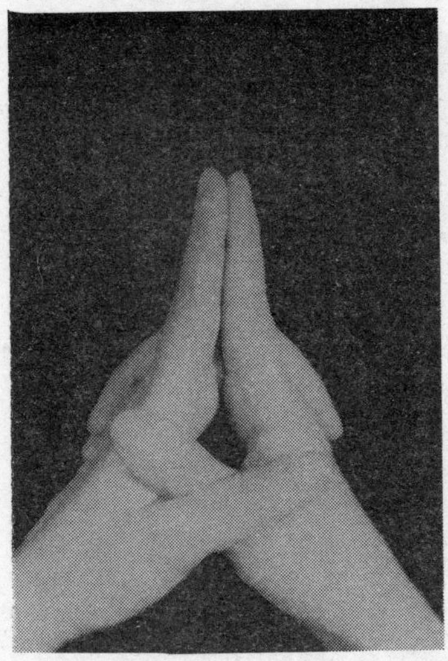

Rebalancing key-ins to the forebrain

(The little fingers, fourth fingers and middle fingers are intertwined externally. The forefingers are extended and held alongside each other. The thumbs are crossed over each other.)

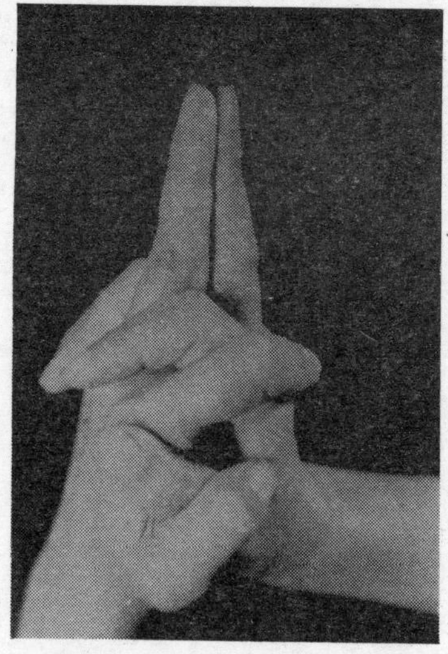

Rebalancing midbrain blocks

(The little fingers, fourth fingers, forefingers and thumbs are externally interlaced. The middle fingers are extended and placed alongside each other.)

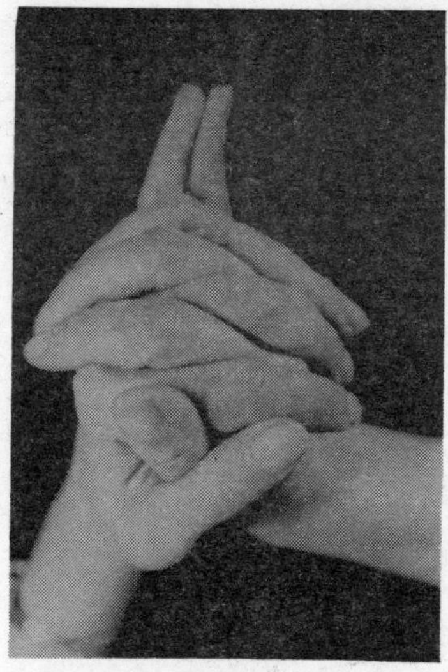

Rebalancing hindbrain blocks

(The fourth fingers, middle fingers, forefingers and thumbs are externally interlaced. The little fingers are extended and placed alongside each other.)

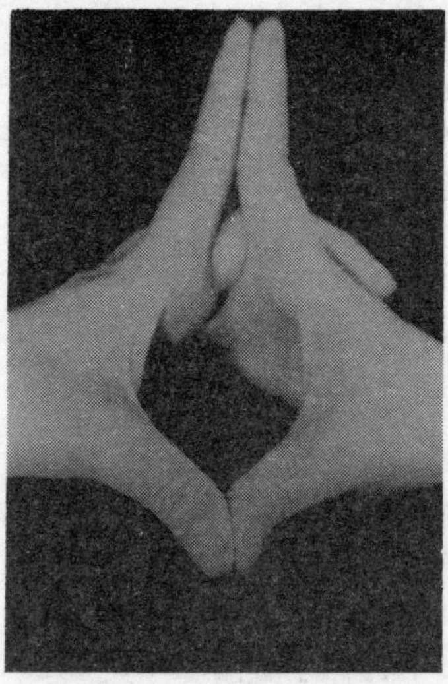

Creating positive energy (1)

With this position, flows are generated which help the self and others in the vicinity to be rebalanced through *foreground* awareness. (The little fingers, fourth fingers and middle fingers are externally interlaced. The forefingers and thumbs are extended in opposite directions, with the tips of the thumbs and the tips of the fingers placed together.)

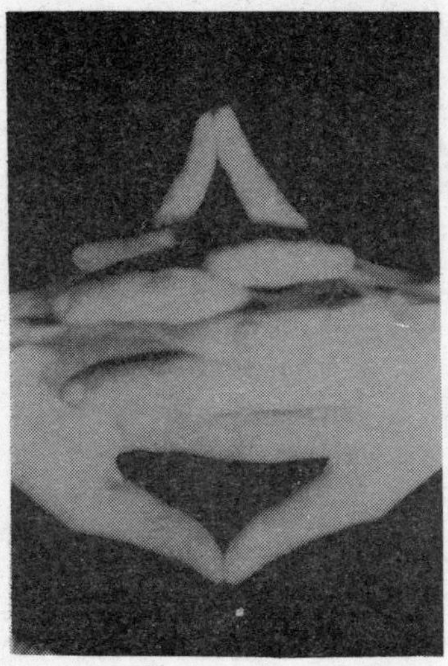

Creating positive energy (2)

This time, flows are generated which help the self and others in the vicinity to be rebalanced through *background* awareness. This position also triggers the flow of key-ins which have become stuck in background awareness. (The fourth fingers, middle fingers and forefingers are externally interlaced. The tips of the little fingers and the tips of the thumbs are brought together.)

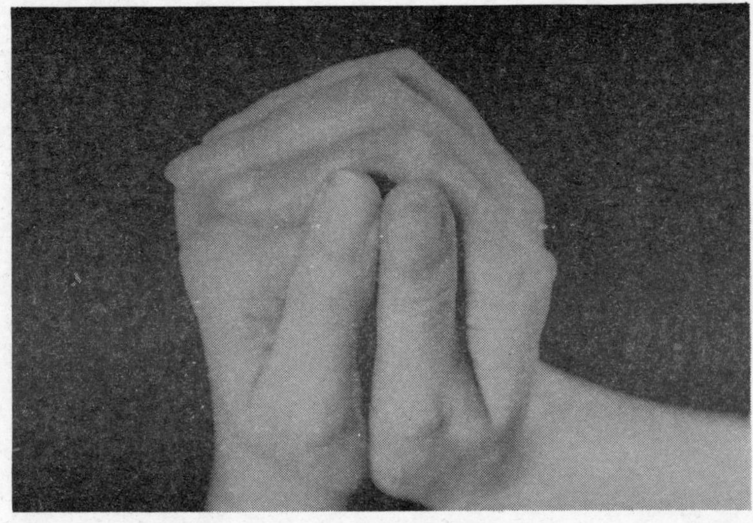

Rebalancing with visualisation wide open

(The closed fist of one hand is covered with the other hand and the two thumbs are held alongside each other.)

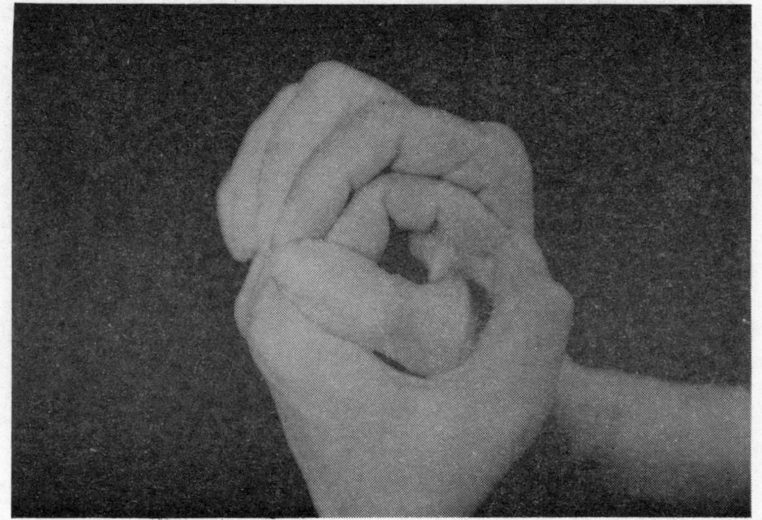

Inside self

(A pair of interlocked chain links are made with the thumbs and forefingers. The remaining fingers of the lower hand are closed to form a fist. The remaining fingers of the upper hand are closed over the lower hand.)

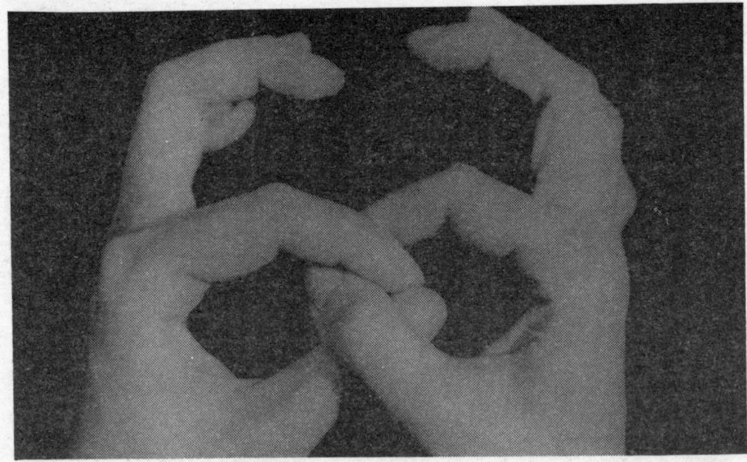

Step 1

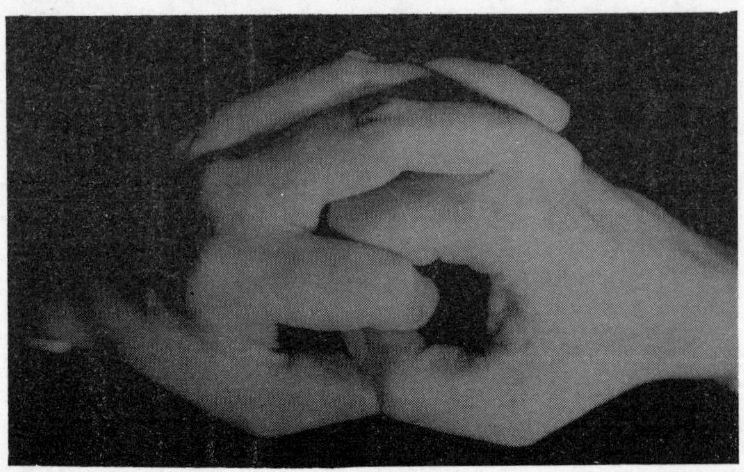

Step 2

Key-ins

(A pair of interlocked chain links are made with the thumb and forefinger of each hand (*Step 1*). The remaining three fingers of each hand are then externally interlinked. The point where the chain links cross is maintained at the tips of the thumbs and forefingers (*Step* 2).)

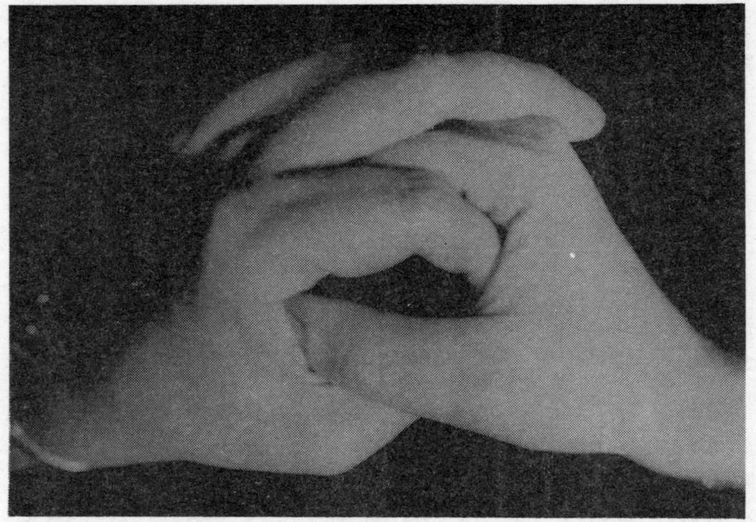

Rebalancing muscle tensions

(Starting from *Step* 2 of the previous position, the hands are brought closer together until the forefinger and thumb of each hand, which still form a chain link, are pushed into close contact with the palm of the opposite hand.)

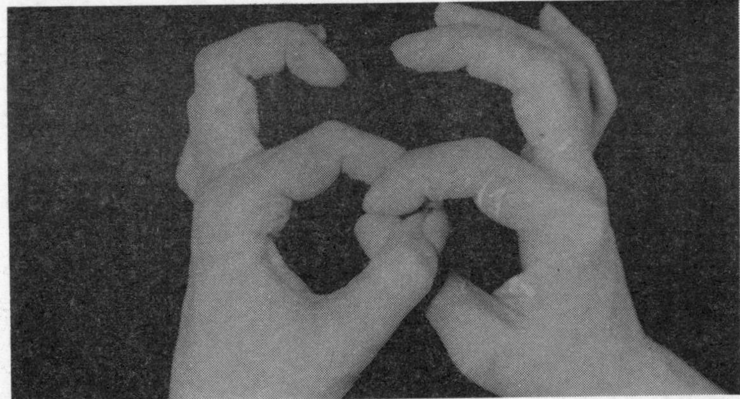

Step 1

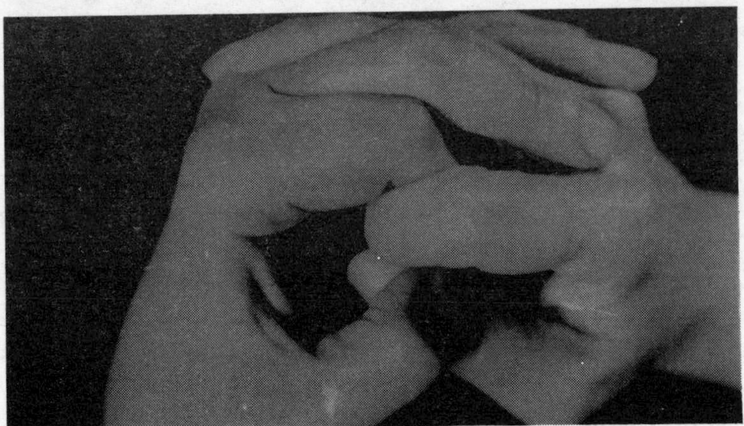

Step 2

Rebalancing natural emotions

This position encourages energies to flow from the body to the mind. (A pair of interlocked chain links is made with the thumbs and forefingers (*Step 1*). The remaining three fingers of each hand are then interlaced in such a way that the middle finger and forefinger of the lower hand come between the middle finger and forefinger of the upper hand. The point where the chain links cross is maintained at the forefinger and thumb tips; all four of these should be in contact with each other (*Step 2*).)

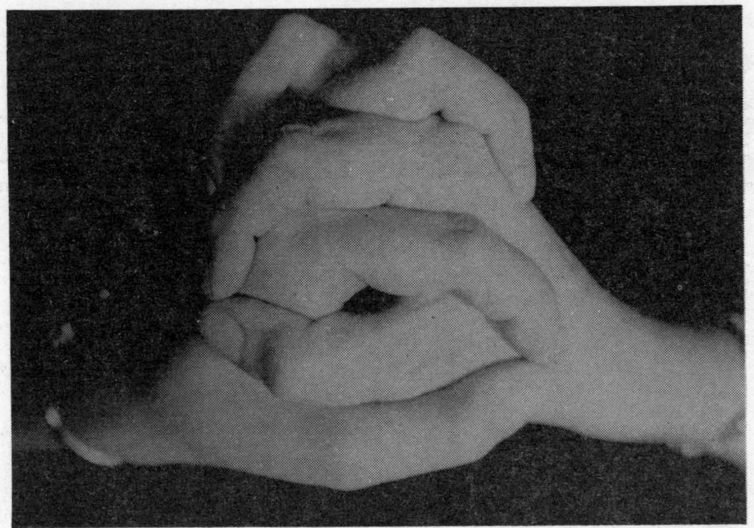

Rebalancing cellular tensions

(Starting from the previous position, the hands are brought closer together until the palms are nearly touching each other. The links made by the thumbs and forefingers are kept closed.)

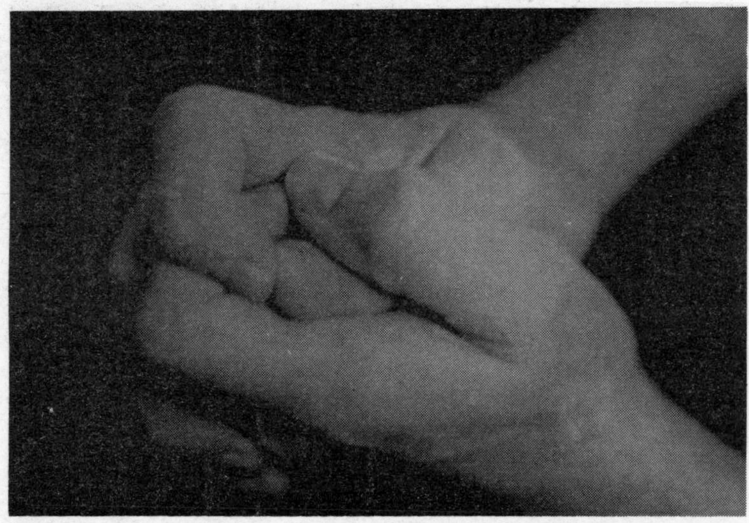

Rebalancing energetic personality affinity

(Starting from previous starting position, the wrists are brought together and the forefinger and thumb chain links, still closed, are lengthened vertically with the knuckle joints squared.)

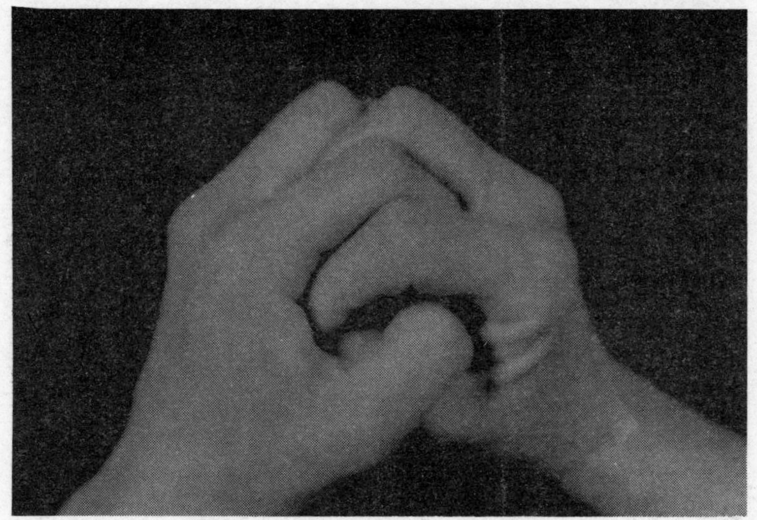

Co-ordinating the two halves of the brain

(All fingers and thumbs are internally interlaced.)

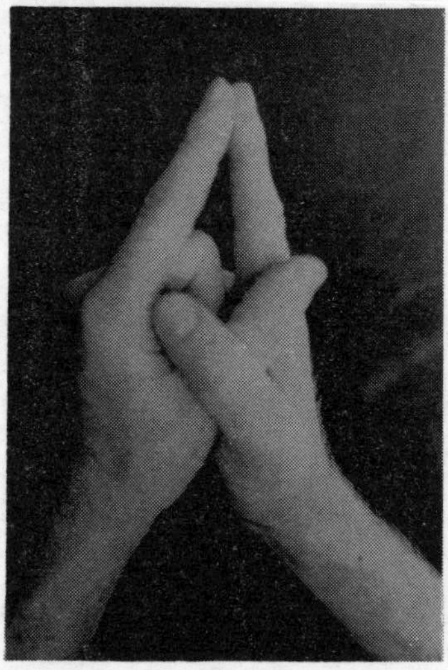

Co-ordinating the neck

(The little fingers, fourth fingers and middle fingers are internally interlaced. The forefingers are extended and made to touch each other at the tips. The thumbs are crossed.)

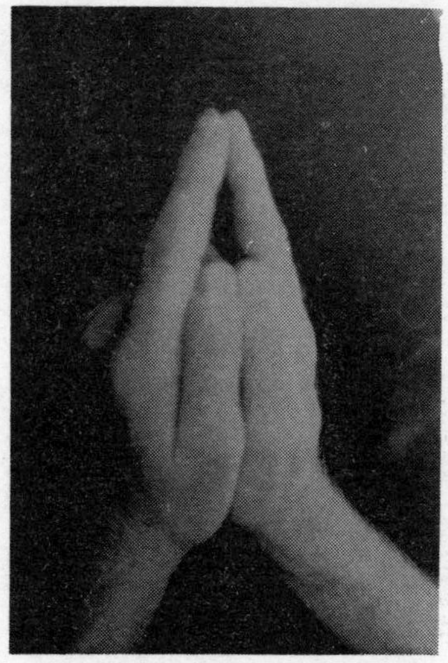

Co-ordinating the backbone

(The little fingers, fourth fingers and middle fingers are internally interlaced. The forefingers and thumbs are extended. The thumbs are held alongside each other and the forefingers touch each other at the tips.)

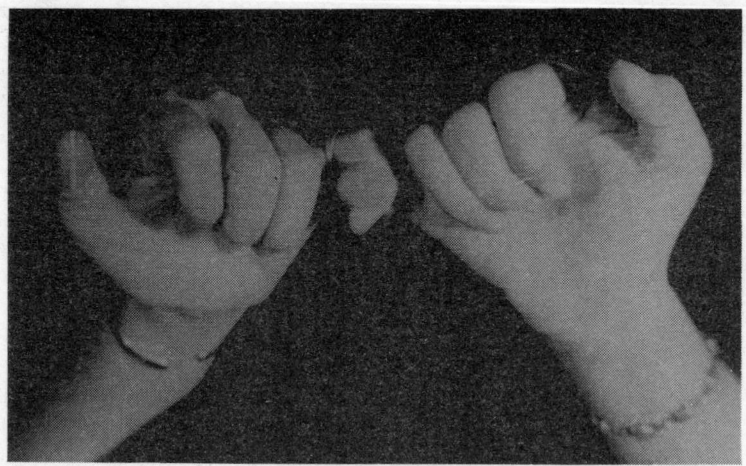

Step 1

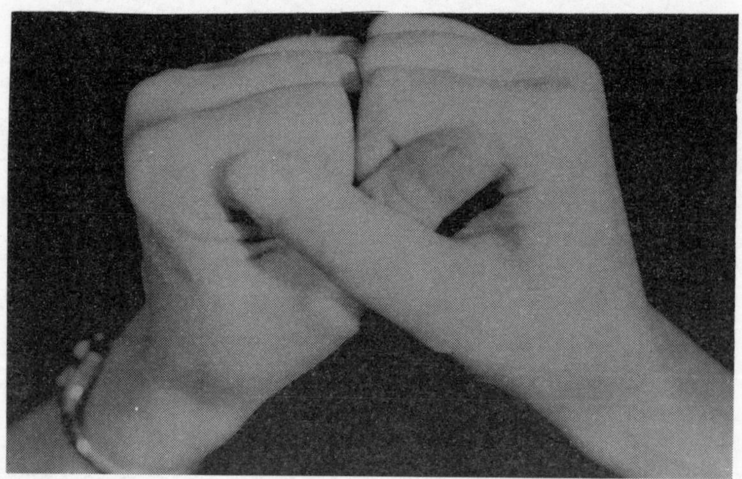

Step 2

Letting go

Rebalancing key-ins are held in place with this position. (The two little fingers are interlocked internally (*Step 1*). The hands are made into fists and brought together with the thumbs crossed over each other (*Step 2*).)

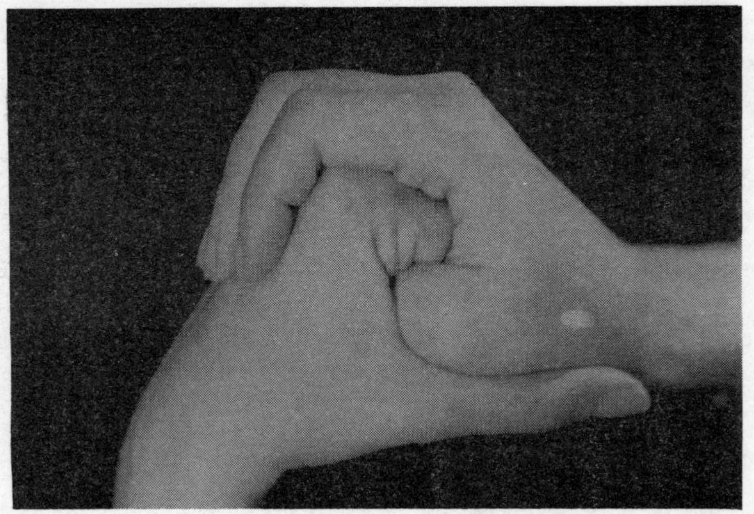

Using outside senses without energy

(The thumb of the outer hand is grasped by the fingers of the inner hand. The fingers of the outer hand cover the inner hand. The thumb of the inner hand lies along the wrist of the outer hand.)

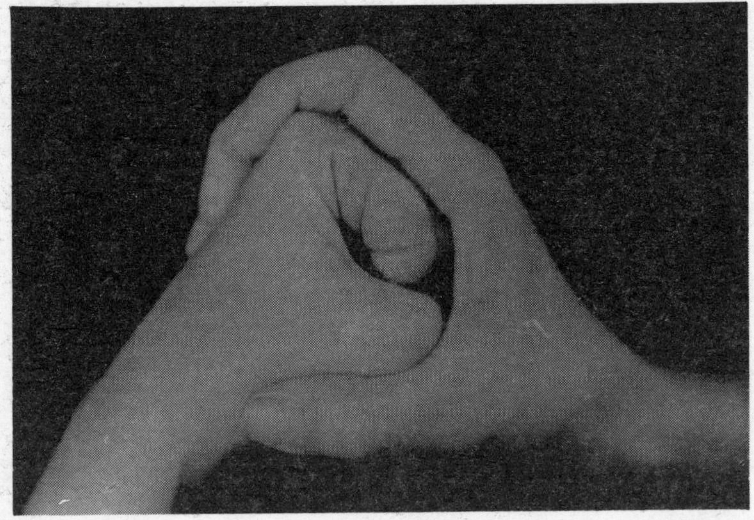

Rebalancing muscle sets

(The closed fist of one hand is grasped between the fingers and thumb of the other hand.)

Rebalancing head blocks

(The thumb of the outer hand is grasped by the fingers of the inner hand. The little finger and fourth finger of the outer hand are closed against the palm of that hand (*Step 1*). The forefinger and middle finger of the outer hand are then closed across the knuckles of the inner hand. The thumb of the inner hand lies along the wrist of the outer hand (*Step* 2).)

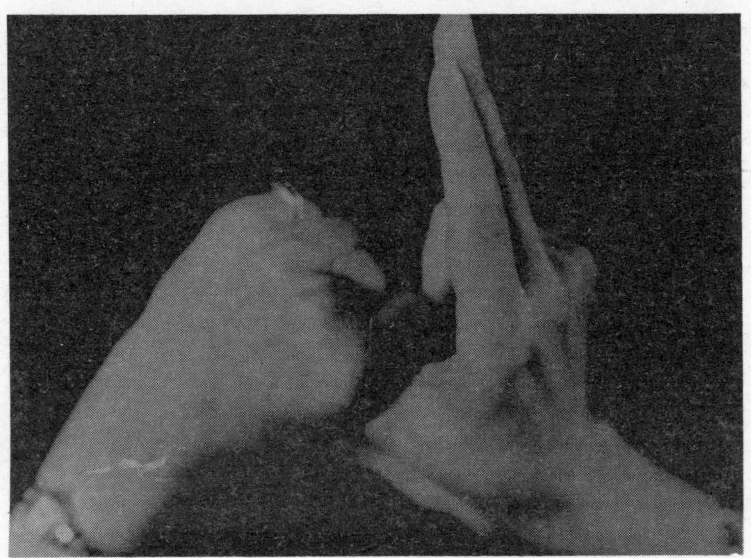

Step 1

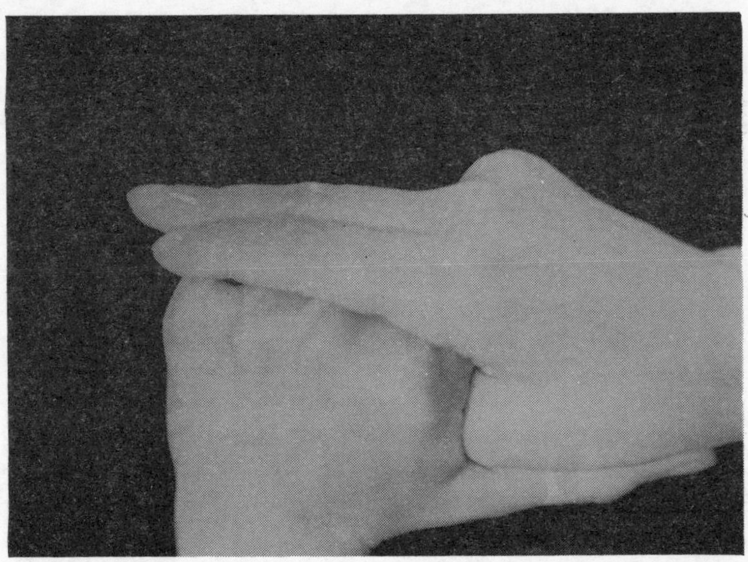

Step 2

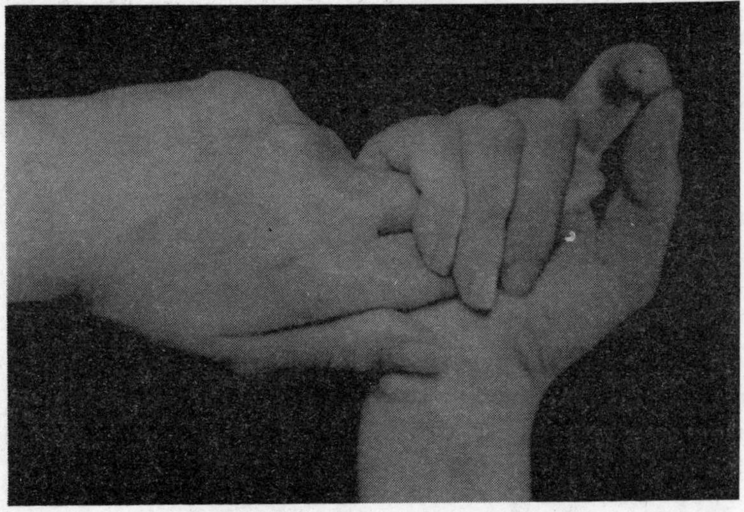

Sharpening the mind for business activity

(The thumb, forefinger and middle finger of the first hand are placed in the palm of the second hand and grasped by the little finger, fourth finger and middle finger of the second hand. A circle is made by bringing together the tips of the forefinger and thumb of the second hand. The little finger and fourth finger of the first hand are closed against the palm of that hand.)

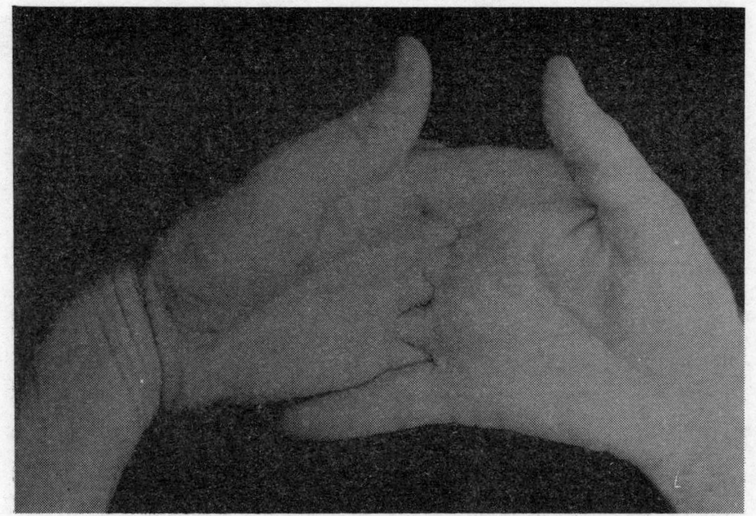

Rebalancing willpower

(Each hand is made into a fist and the two wrists are crossed at right angles so as to touch each other on the inside.)

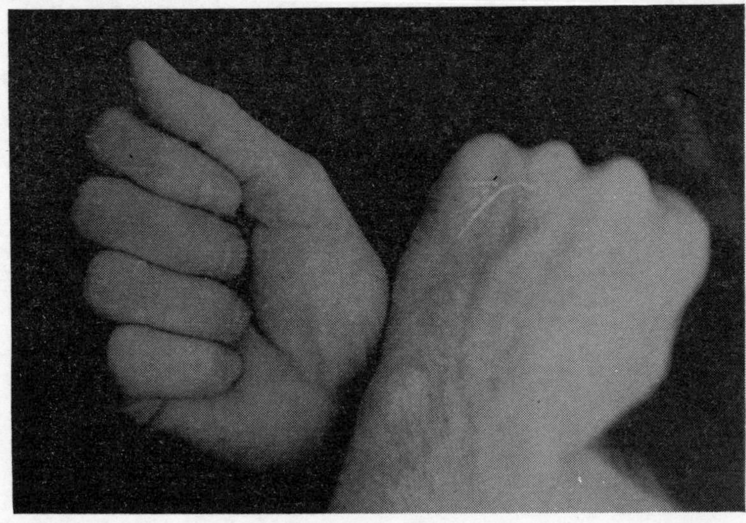

Inducing relaxation

(The fingers, but not the thumbs, are externally interlaced. The combined palms are then placed over the body part that requires to be relaxed, for example the eyes, forehead, or jaws.)

7

Energy in Bones and Muscles

WHEN ISAAC NEWTON discovered the law of gravity, he was totally unaware that this very same law was a major contributor to the ills of man. Gravity starts to pull the human structure out of balance from the time we are an embryo until the day we go to the grave. Much as an unbalanced wheel will cause a watch to stop or an unbalanced load will cause a ship to capsize, so an unbalanced body will cause innumerable ailments in the human being.

George Ivan Carter, through years of study and inspiration, has developed a simple, foolproof method of realigning the body structure and it is by these means that the human body may be brought into perfect balance and thus back to perfect health and normal operation. He had come to the conclusion that in order to have harmony, peace of mind and health within the human body, perfect balance must be maintained in all the bones and joints.

This original and scientific system has proved itself to be effective over the past few decades. Testimonies from thousands of people tell of the marvellous results it has had in helping to relieve the suffering of humanity.

Carter worked closely with my friend Leonard Allan, who in turn has instructed me in the relevant techniques and who has kindly given me permission to use his material.

The method of letting the body's own energy do the necessary work is a pleasure to witness, as no force is used at any time. The simple formula used is that of holding the opposites. For example, if one bone or area has dropped due to an energy pull, this ought to be held from underneath: usually the thumb or fingers are to be placed uppermost on the opposite side — this hold allows the body energy to benefit the patient.

Unfortunately, the "stress of life" affects the nervous system, the blood system and also the muscles of the body, which register this stress through "tension". Very few of us pay any attention to our posture. However, bad posture will produce a marked distortion and this in turn will cause certain pressures which will restrict the blood flow and ultimately the nervous function of the body.

If people would only realise what misery and distress is caused to the human body by the mastoids and the neck being out of position! The neck sometimes becomes very stiff and sore, and if the middle bone of the neck is pulled out of alignment, this interferes with the teeth by cutting off the circulation and nerve energy, causing the teeth to decay and the gums to become infected.

The first step in rebuilding the body structure is to consider the neck and shoulders. If the neck is seen to be crooked and the shoulders out of alignment, then this will have affected the position of the internal organs.

The shoulder blades are responsible for the condition of the neck. If the right shoulder is lower and appears to be longer than the left one, you will find that the left shoulder blade will be an inch higher than the right one. If you then examine the back of the shoulder, you will feel a large solid lump. The right shoulder blade will have moved down and there will be very little tension, if any, above the shoulder blade. The right shoulder blade will crowd the spine out of position towards the left, or closer to the left shoulder blade. This will cause the seventh cervical, or the large bone on the back of the neck, to move to the left also. The cervical region, or the neck bones, will be drawn to the right and cause the atlas, or top bone of the neck, to twist out of position.

By closely examining the front of the neck, you will find that the right side of the neck seems to be a trifle larger and firmer. This is the starting point for trouble with your eyes, ears, nose and mouth, as well as migraine headaches. Your chest will become prominent, or very full, on the left side, while on the right side a depression will become noticeable which will interfere with your breathing. Such cases have been termed tuberculosis of the lungs. The reverse condition of the chest would indicate a wheezing or asthma.

It is obvious to anyone who tries it that when one stands with the left shoulder lowered, the spine will move to a different position. Again, when the left shoulder is raised, the opposite one drops. Doing this gives a quick and clear understanding of how the spine will move from one position to the other and how rigid the ligaments will become inside the body under the higher shoulder and how the opposite side will become so relaxed that it forces the internal organs of the body to move out of place and become congested.

If distortion is present, especially in the head area, different parts of the body begin to move out of shape. A twist in the neck or shoulders, pulling them out of alignment, may interfere with the entire nervous system. Once a disturbance in the autonomous nervous system has been triggered, then the whole body will produce some peculiar and dangerous symptoms which are normally, although wrongly, termed a disease.

I do not intend to present a resumé of the working of the nervous system — this knowledge can be gained from books in any library. Nevertheless, I hope your interest will be aroused and that you will endeavour to learn more about the workings of the body.

The complications produced by any distortion caused by

an energy pull has far-reaching implications. The glandular or endocrine systems can even be affected. One must be aware that the human frame always presents a clear picture of the individual who owns that frame and must be observed in this context. Blood pressures can be helped by means of such observation and the application of the methods described later in the chapter.

In a roundabout way, distortion of the human frame does affect the lymphatic drainage, which is even more important to the body than the blood flow. Very little has been written on this subject, so please bear with me while I attempt to explain its significance.

The lymphatic system is of great importance. The lymphatic vessels are far greater in number than the arteries and veins, and have connections with all parts of the internal organs. They are to be found in the skin of the body, face and scalp, and have a great influence on the thyroid gland. They carry the sense action to all parts of our body. If the lymphatic system is not functioning efficiently, the sense of taste, for example, will be diminished. The lymph also has a great influence on the action or movement of any part of the neck and hands. If the lymph becomes thick and sluggish, it gradually slows up the action of the blood, as the glands supply strength to the red blood cells. The more active the lymph becomes, the more quickly the body will move.

The lymphatic system consists of a complex network of connecting vessels, which collect the lymph from the various organs and tissues of the body and conduct it to the large veins of the neck, connecting with the jugular vein and veins of less importance, where the lymph is poured into the bloodstream. In this system of connecting vessels there are many lymph glands or nodes; these little nodes or sacs, acting as filters and separating one substance from another, resemble buttons on a string and are placed at different distances apart.

In order to examine this system in greater detail we will start with the head and face. We will draw an imaginary line from the back of the throat to meet with the third cervical (the bone in the middle of the neck). Here we find these strings of lymphatic nodes coming out from the deeper tissues and travelling through the flesh on the face and head beneath the skin; one branch occupies the skin and travels up the jaw to the eyes, while two other branches travel to the nose. The important nodes lie between the ear and the cheek bone, along a line from the ear to the tip of the nose. From here the strings of glands, fifteen or twenty in number, travel up both sides of the head. The function of these glands is to collect fats and waste materials and carry them into the deeper portions of the body. Just above the collar bone on either side of the neck we find a group of these little nodes, five or six on either side extending down into the deeper part of the body, and branches extend down through the flesh and connect with the shoulders. You can feel these little nodes in many parts of the body.

The next group is located in the back of the neck, and travels up inside the skull, forming a drainage system for different parts, and continues from there down to the extreme lower part of the body. The heat ratio of our body depends greatly on the action of these lymphatic nodes.

Now we will direct our attention to the lymphatic system of the neck, which starts beneath the chin and travels along the two main arteries down to the breast bone (sternum). One group of lymphatics, which again appear as buttons on a string, can be found descending from the collar bone to the solar plexus. There is also a little string of lymph nodes or buttons that seems to extend from the spinal column, sending out branches to the various parts of the flesh and diaphragm.

If we go back to just below the collar bone, we find a large knot with branches running in different directions, travelling down beneath the flesh and extending into the armpit. From there, many lymphatic veins travel down the arm on both sides, but the largest group inhabits the palms of the hands and the fingers. It is here that we can notice most clearly the relation between the lymphatic system and the conscious system, which carries the sense vibration of our body. All that you need to do to trace the lymphatics is to draw the finger of your right hand along the corresponding finger on the left hand and you will experience the great sensation of touch.

The next group of lymphatics extends from the shoulders, and in this case is seated deeper in the flesh, extending down the trunk of the body, with branches going to the breast. The entire breast is one solid network of glands, with the exception of the nipple. This network of lymphatics has a strong influence on the mammary glands.

In the lower part of the back (the lumbar region) we find a large lymphatic gland similar to an artery. At this point the gland branches out and has many nodes, a dozen or so. Other little strings of nodes extend down into the lower part of the body to the fallopian tubes, ovarian glands, uterus, vagina and lower limbs. These glands collect the lymph from the lower extremities and carry it in the direction of the heart. There it connects with one of the main arteries and pours the lymph and chyle (a milk-like substance) into the blood. The lymph is carried around by the circulation of the blood until the blood passes through the kidneys, where the detrimental substance is extracted from the blood and then eliminated by the force of the urinary channels.

To take you a step further to the understanding of the far-reaching healing effects of the lymphatic system, I will mention a little more about the skull and facial bones, before moving on to explain the importance of the mastoid bones.

Skull and Facial Bones

The bones of the skull can move out of position through many causes. First let us consider the jawbone: if the left side of the skull is low, the right side will be forced out of position. This will cause the teeth on the left side of the mouth to close much more firmly than on the right side, and then we will be inclined to chew our food on the left side of the mouth. By doing this we will take the pressure off the teeth on the right side, which stop the nerve action and the circulation of the blood to both the upper and lower teeth on that side of the face. In many cases this leads to ulcers of the teeth, toothache or a condition of pyorrhoea. Moreover, if the lower jawbone is low, then the cheek bone will also be lower. This causes the sinus and facial bone to become twisted out of shape. This unnatural pressure on the facial bones will also cause problems in the antrums, or with the adenoids, causing a blockage in the sinuses.

By standing before the mirror and placing one finger of the right hand under the right cheek bone and one finger of the left hand under the left cheek bone, we can tell just how much the facial bones have moved out of position.

In a close examination of the bones of your face, one eye will frequently appear to be lower than the other. This is just the case when the facial bones are out of position. Then the frontal or forehead bone will show the same indication; the bone of the forehead having moved down the left side causes the left eye also to be lower. As the left side of the frontal part of the skull moves downwards, this naturally causes the back of the skull on the same side to move upwards. This movement will interfere with the position of the mastoid gland, bringing an unnatural pressure to bear on the medulla and interfering with the senses of sight and hearing, as the mastoid bone will have been made to rise, corresponding with the back of the skull.

Such movement of the skull and facial bones will prevent the head from sitting in a straight position upon the atlas (the top bone of the spine), thus causing pressure on the nerves of the spine, and leading to a lack of energy in the brain, eyes, ears, nose and throat. Thus, to a certain extent, the circulation to the different parts of the head and face is restricted.

In many cases, people who are not sure of their step will occasionally stumble and fall or their ankle will turn; this too is caused by pressure on the brain. Again, we notice people who at times stagger, or are afraid to go up to high elevations, or to climb a ladder to unreasonable heights, and look down from the top of high buildings exclaiming, "Oh, this makes me dizzy". Now, the cause of all this interference is located in the brain, directly under the temporal bone which is just above the ear. The left side of the forehead being low, a pressure is exerted on this bone, crowding it in and in turn bringing a pressure on the brain. This same bone on the opposite side of the head will protrude causing fullness on the right side of the head and contributing to the pressure on the centre of balance in the brain. This pressure not only causes the troubles mentioned above, but it also unbalances man's whole system — his thinking, his will and the action of the entire body.

If the skull is higher on one side than the other, the resulting pressure on the brain will stop the effective function of this portion of the brain and the nervous system that connects with some of the vital parts of our body. The skull moving out of position many times is often responsible for the appearance of lymphatic tumours in the scalp.

If the forehead is out of alignment, with one side higher than the other, you will clearly notice this in the bony structure above the eyes. If there is a depression in the skull, just to the back of the forehead, this will cause the neck to become stiff, the shoulders to move out of alignment, and significant problems will arise in the hands and wrists.

At the top of the skull, on each side of the centre point, there is a direct connection between the underlying portion of the brain and the feet, especially the toes and metatarsal arches.

If a defect appears at the back of the skull, we may experience problems with both the eyes and ears. Misplaced bones in this area of the skull cause pressure on the brain or the cells of the brain that connect with different parts of our body.

Finally, there is an opening in the top of our skull through which we make spiritual contact with the conscious system. Again, any displacement of the bones will affect our ability to maintain this contact.

Having considered the various sections of the skull that might become displaced, and the great influence and pressure that will be brought to bear on the nerves and circulation of the head and face, and on different sections of the brain, it will now be clear that it may take a number of treatments to realign the skull into a perfect condition and relieve the nerves and the circulation of the blood.

The Mastoid Bones and Glands

The mastoid bones, or processes, are located just behind the ears and continue back along the base of the skull, between the temporal and occipital bones. They have a direct effect on our ability to hear. As do the other divisions of the skull, the mastoids sometimes move out of position and cause considerable problems with the hearing. If the left side of the skull moves forward, this will interfere with the hearing of the left ear, with the associated problem of dry wax. A parallel disturbance on the right side of the skull will have the same effect on the right ear.

We tend not to pay much attention to the mastoid bones, but when we do stop to consider them we find that they are a process of much importance, as we find inside them air chambers similar to the sinuses in the frontal part of the head. The interior of the lower part of the mastoid bones consists of small cells resembling those of a honeycomb. These cells contain marrow and different kinds of hormones which provide lubrication for the ear. Later, these become a waxy substance. In cases where the red blood is interfered with, or where the circulation is restricted, the heat ratio in the mastoids and ears will decrease. The shell, or the outside of the mastoid bones is almost as hard as ivory.

The two mastoid bones are connected by tissue. This tissue extends forward, making a connection with the inner eardrum. The outer eardrums, both right and left, make connection with the mastoid glands, which are located directly behind them. These glands are not as noticeable in children as they are in older people.

If there is an interference in the ears caused by the mastoid glands, our senses of sight, taste and smell will also be affected. In the case where the skull is deformed or out of alignment, pressure will be brought to bear on the mastoid glands, interfering with the medulla, and also affecting the senses of taste and smell. The seat of sight is located in the back of the head, also near the mastoid bones. Therefore, if there is an unnatural pressure on these bones, the effectiveness of the person's sight will be diminished.

In many cases of an eruption in the mastoid bone, a fever or inflammation may appear. This causes the bone behind the ear to become sore and, in turn, the mastoid glands to become enlarged, with detrimental consequences for the tongue and the throat. One gland from each mastoid extends down the throat and is attached to the collar bone. A feverish condition of the mastoid may therefore result in many disorders and throat problems, causing large deposits of phlegm or mucus in the throat. You may recognise these conditions by the very bad odour noticeable from the nostrils.

There is also another connection to the mastoid — a small acute gland travelling upwards close behind the ear. This has often been referred to as an inferior duct and in many cases will have been surgically removed. However, the removal of this little gland or duct may have serious repercussions for the brain, as blood poisoning sometimes develops in the mastoid. It should always be remembered that the position of the back of the skull has a great influence on the mastoid bones and glands.

George Ivan Carter was rich in his knowledge of the body, but not in the mundane sense. He had something that was inexplicable, yet very ordinary in application. He often expressed himself in simple ways, yet he was always profound. He did say that every organ of the body will indicate its condition by a symptom.

When a problem occurs in the eyes, ears, throat or other organ, you will find cold spots on the head, the back of the neck, the shoulders and arms, and above the location area of each organ of the body, for each organ of the body perspires just as the brow does, and if for any reason the perspiration is checked, a cold spot develops. For example, if the liver is not working properly, there will be a cold spot over the liver as the relevant sweat glands will cease to function. As the perspiration leaves the body in other areas, you will notice an odour specific to the retarded action of the liver. At other times, the odour of the body may point to a malfunction in the stomach and bowel, or in the kidneys.

You can locate the cause of the trouble yourself by passing the palms of the hands over the flesh. When you come to a cold spot, you will know that the organ directly beneath it needs attention. If the gall bladder is impaired, or the gall duct, you will find the cold spot located on the right side of your body just at the bottom of the diaphragm near the bottom of the ribs. Your spleen is also of importance. You will find the cold spot for the pancreas and the spleen on the opposite side of the body — at the left side — just at the bottom of the ribs. Place your hand on the ribs when you treat the pancreas and spleen.

If the cause of your distress lies in the respiratory system, then right at the end of the breast bone you will find the centre for the solar plexus, which will take care of your breathing problems in a very short time. You must understand that this great nerve centre of the body, called a plexus, connects groups of nerves extending to all organs of the body, and when you treat your body from this centre you will immediately feel the warmth of the minerals passing into your body, into each and every organ.

As has been noted earlier, our thinking faculties are divided into three separate parts: objective, subjective and subconscious. Our thinking is transferred from the Universal Mind to the three divisions of our brain. Our thoughts, actions and deeds depend greatly upon the action of our conscious system, upon our brain. If the organism of our body is not functioning properly, then the communications from the conscious system to our brain are interfered with, causing heavy, sluggish thinking. A torpid liver, gall bladder trouble, constipation and many other ailments interfere with our consciousness and detract from the efficient action of the brain.

In this study of brain, mind and thought, we will see many different bodily influences that can and will interfere with our thinking.

Various parts of our body have a direct connection with the brain. Thus, a disarranged skull may interfere with any natural talent that humanity is entitled to exercise. If the temple division of the skull is out of position, this will be very easily detected by moving your hands slowly over the skull. You will discover a groove in the skull or that its surface is uneven. If the parietal bones bulge on either side, this will cause pressure on the nervous system of the entire body, causing a person to experience worry or fear. If the frontal bones have moved far enough out of position to bring a pressure on the frontal part of the brain, this interferes with the intelligence. If the lower division of the skull in the back of the head (occipital) moves downward in the slightest degree, then the resulting pressure on the mastoid gland will interfere with the hearing. This same condition may also cause serious eye strain. Now, if these pressures are also brought to bear on the different parts of the brain, the effect will be an interference with our thinking process.

If we have a correct understanding of our thinking and hearing, we can use the mind to a greater extent. As I have said, there is but one mind — the Universal Mind — which passes through the three divisions of our brain. If our brain is clear of bodily pressures and the nervous system is free of interference, we can translate the Universal Mind into very valuable thinking, as the mind passes through the translator, which is located in the frontal part of our head. We may translate from this mind some very valuable thoughts, which will bring to us information that we may have been seeking for years. Many things that seem to be confusing and hard to understand will be made plain to us by clear thinking. But the essential prerequisite for clear thinking is clear action of the brain.

In order to have this clear action, we must have a clear brain. Finally, it follows that in order to have a clear brain, we must have a body that is functioning properly, free from aches and pains, free from constipation and inefficient digestion. Our lymphatic system must work properly. The flesh and skin must carry out their functions without interference. Our conscious system must be free from depression, our liver, gall bladder, pancreas and spleen must function properly. We must have a reconnection of our body, our soul and our spirit; then we can think correctly, both physically and spiritually. We should be very careful when we are translating the mind into thought.

It is a well-established fact that a single diagram is worth a thousand words. No effort has been spared to give you many explicit instructions in the diagrams which follow. It is hoped that you will be able to use these to help you to bring your body back to perfect balance. We will begin with an introduction to George Ivan Carter's method for aligning the bones in the body, looking in particular at the mastoid bones. Next, we will look at the various specific contact points on different areas of the body. These contact points are the ones to be used when working through the holds or moves illustrated in the rest of the chapter.

Aligning the Body: The Mastoid Bone

George Ivan Carter always stressed that the mastoid bone is the springboard to health. His system of healing depends on adjusting all the bones in the body. According to Carter, when Newton discovered the law of gravity, he missed something very important. It is "gravity" which is responsible for man's ills; gravity pulls man's entire physical structure out of balance.

What happens to the human head is very important because it encompasses the human brain. It is seldom that one will find a perfectly balanced head, thus there is not a bone that is correctly balanced.

Most of us have a displaced mastoid bone and this is evident by observing that one side of the head is lower than the other. Carter's process of aligning all these misplaced bones is a fairly complex operation, involving about 400 movements which will eventually align the whole body. The diagrams below show two of the most important ones, the first one for aligning the mastoid bones and the second for aligning the upper scapula.

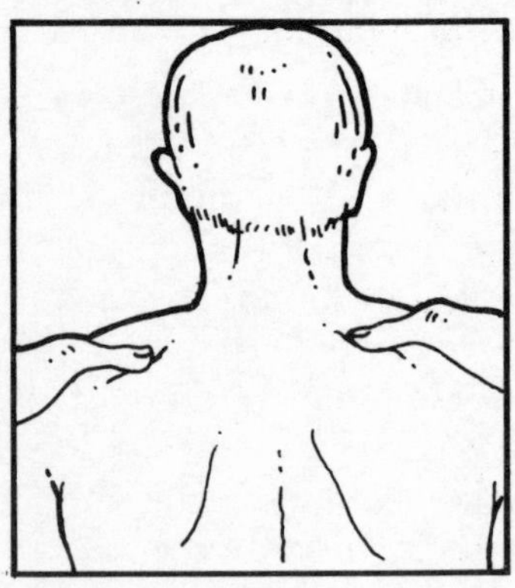

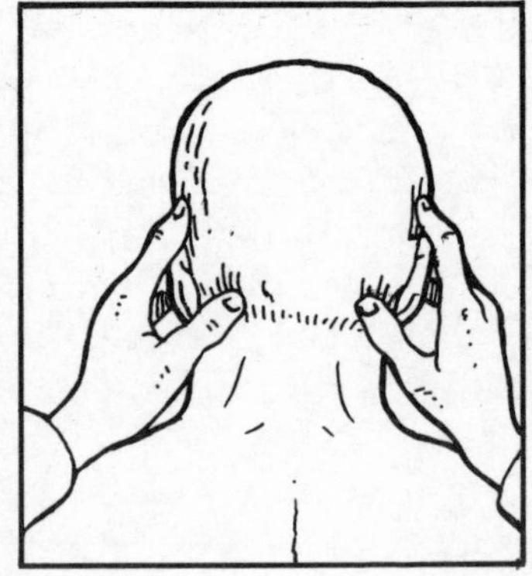

Facial Contacts
It will be observed that contact points are to be found practically all over the facial area. The width of the touch to use is about that of the tip of an index finger. The pressures exerted should be very light — no pushing or massaging.

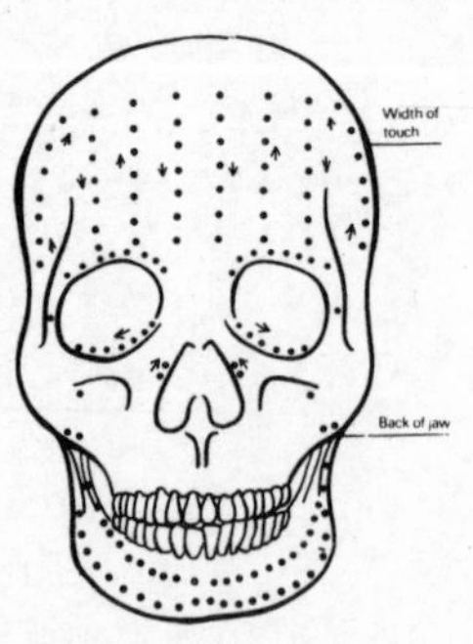

Head Contacts

These contact points are on the posterior of the head. One may view these contacts as the main control areas for restoring equilibrium to the head. The action of balancing these contacts by gentle touch has deep ramifications, especially with the lower points on the bottom of the head, known as the Nuchal Zone, so do be gentle.

Don't let it worry you if you are unsure of how to locate the contacts. The more you use your powers of observation, the more the contact areas will become apparent.

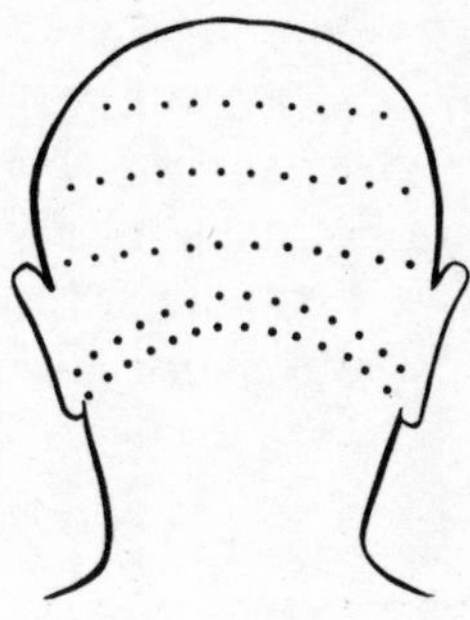

Malar Bone Contacts

On each side of the face is a long bone extending from the ear to the nose. This is called the Zygomatic bone. The balance of these areas affects the whole skull area and also the eye sockets. You will observe there are some contact points above and some below this bone area.

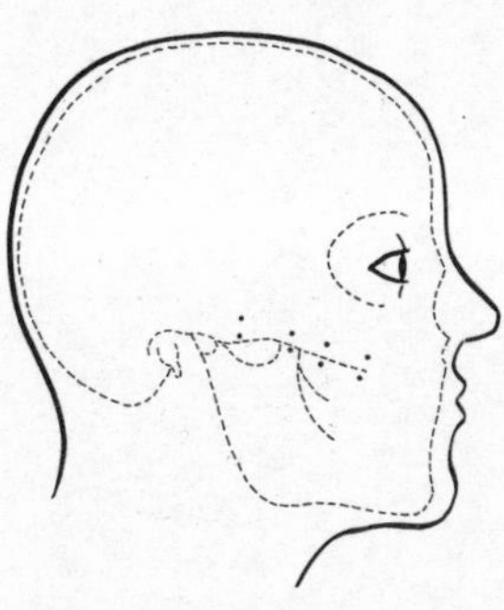

A slight touch-hold above or below is all that is required. The results are fantastic if both sides are balanced. Observe the high side and the low side. Place the index finger under the low side and the other index finger above the high side; just hold and feel it balance. Headaches will melt away with these simple contacts.

Anterior Body Contacts

Always remember that these areas of joint or bone contact are bilateral (i.e. applying to both sides of the body).

Later in this chapter you will be shown the actual holds to use: some using only the fingers, some using the palms and others using the whole hand.

The joint areas are the most important for the release of energy. Energy usually stagnates in the joints if these are out of balance, resulting in pain and inflammation. Painful and inflamed areas will usually respond favourably, as it is only by a touch-hold that the energy is released.

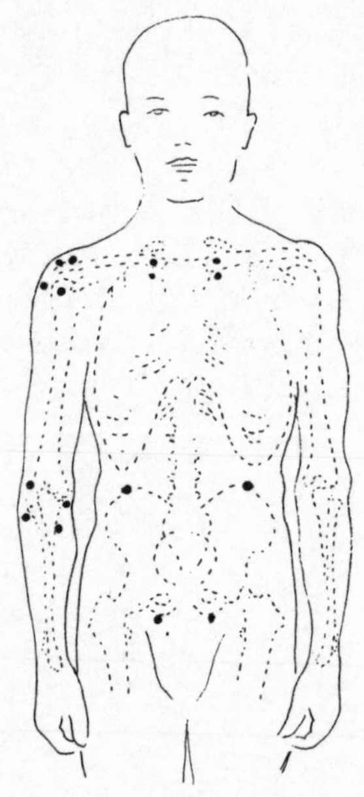

Posterior Body Contacts

There are numerous areas of the back, or posterior, of the body that need balancing by this touch method. Always keep in mind that the contacts are very light, i.e. *no massage* is required, and that both sides of the body should usually be treated.

On the top left of the diagram is shown a gentle stretch-hold for the shoulder if it is painful. Again, it is stressed that this is only a gentle hold — no pulling. Usually, both shoulders should be relaxed by this method.

On the lower corners of the diagram one will observe the simple holds that are applied to the wrist area. there are eight bones which form the wrist, each of which should be held lightly as shown. Always treat both wrists.

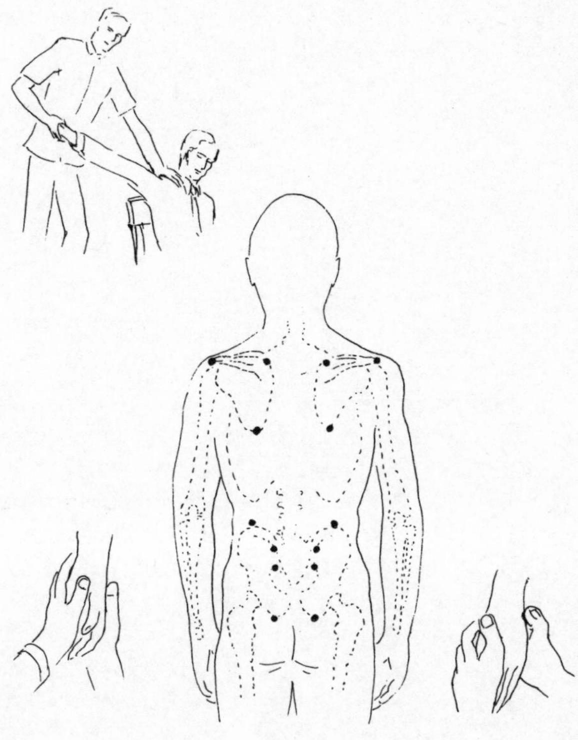

Arm Contacts (Bilateral)
This diagram shows an enlarged version of the contact areas for the shoulder, and also for the elbows.

Usually, in the elbow area both sides of the arm should be balanced. Observation will show if there is any distortion.

The general rule is to touch-hold under the lower bone and above the higher bone. This approach applies to all joints.

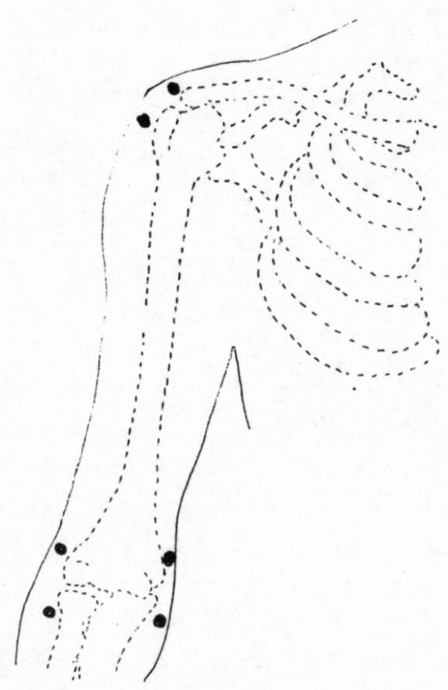

Lower Limb Contacts
The feet are the base of the entire body structure and their balance must be maintained at all costs.

In the top diagrams the contacts used to balance the heels and ankle bones are indicated. It will also be observed that the very bottom of the foot is important; a slip of the cuboid bone will distort the whole foot and thus affect the whole body structure.

Contacts are also shown for the ankle areas and the knees. Painful knees will also have the effect of throwing the hips out of balance.

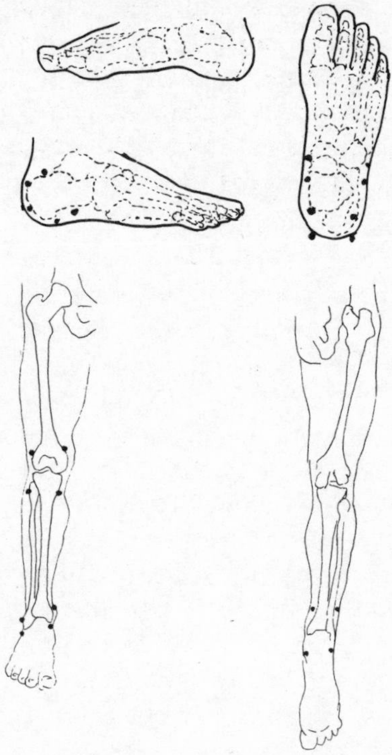

Healing Touches
The diagrams included in the rest of this chapter depict some of the touch-holds that can be done using the contact points already given.

The first series of thirty pictures, which concentrate on the head, will give you a very good idea of what can be achieved, as this method produces different results in various areas.

Always observe the lower side — the high side — the tilted side — the rotated side. By these series of holds and touches, we are aiming to produce a symmetry in the area of operation.

Study each of these thirty illustrations before progressing to those which follow. They will provide a firm basis for your "healing" applications.

Another series of diagrams (31-72) will show you some of the holds or moves used to produce symmetry in the head, the neck, the shoulders and various other parts of the body. It was felt that these simple sketches would give you a clearer understanding of what is required than could volumes of words, which could so easily be misinterpreted.

Normally, one commences by restoring the symmetry of the mastoid bones — then the top of the head — the occipital ridge of the skull — the eye sockets — the malar bones — the nose — the neck. Never be in a hurry, as energy cannot be hurried but only assisted. Then one works the back spinal areas — the chest and rib cage — the pelvis — the hip joints. Then work the elbows — the wrists — the knees — the ankles — the feet, etc. Whichever way you decide to progress the main idea is to produce balance in the body, so one must work through the areas of the body in a systematic way.

Nothing could be more truthful than to tell you that your hands are your fortune. Use them purposefully and use them knowledgeably. Direct your thoughts to the end result you want to accomplish. It is said that "miracles take longer", but by using your hands you have the ability to bring them about *now!*

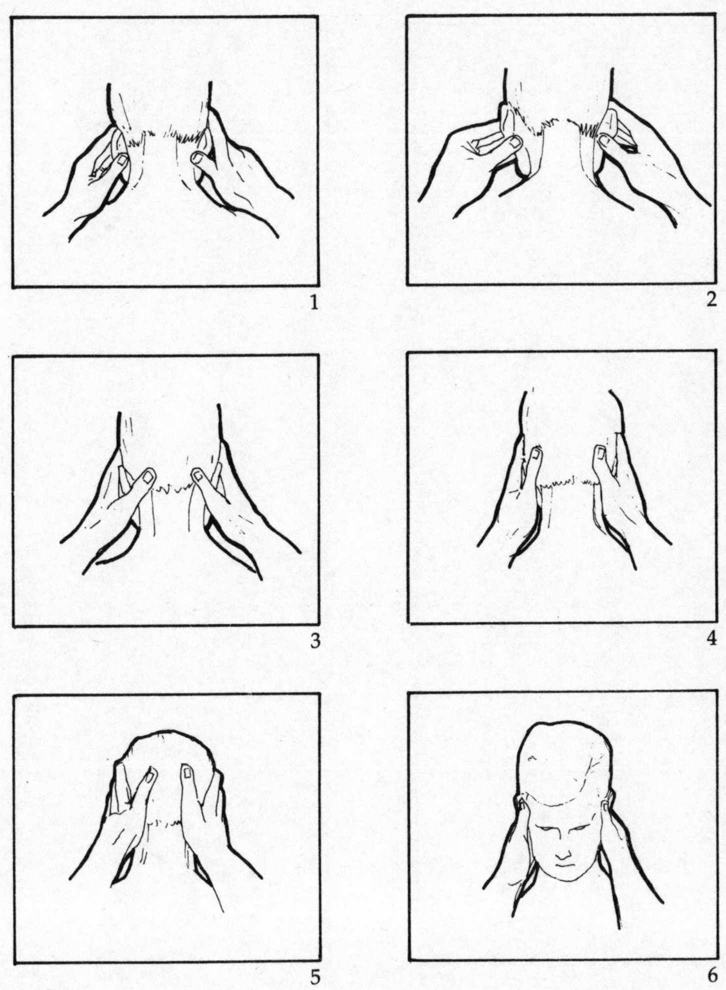
1
2
3
4
5
6

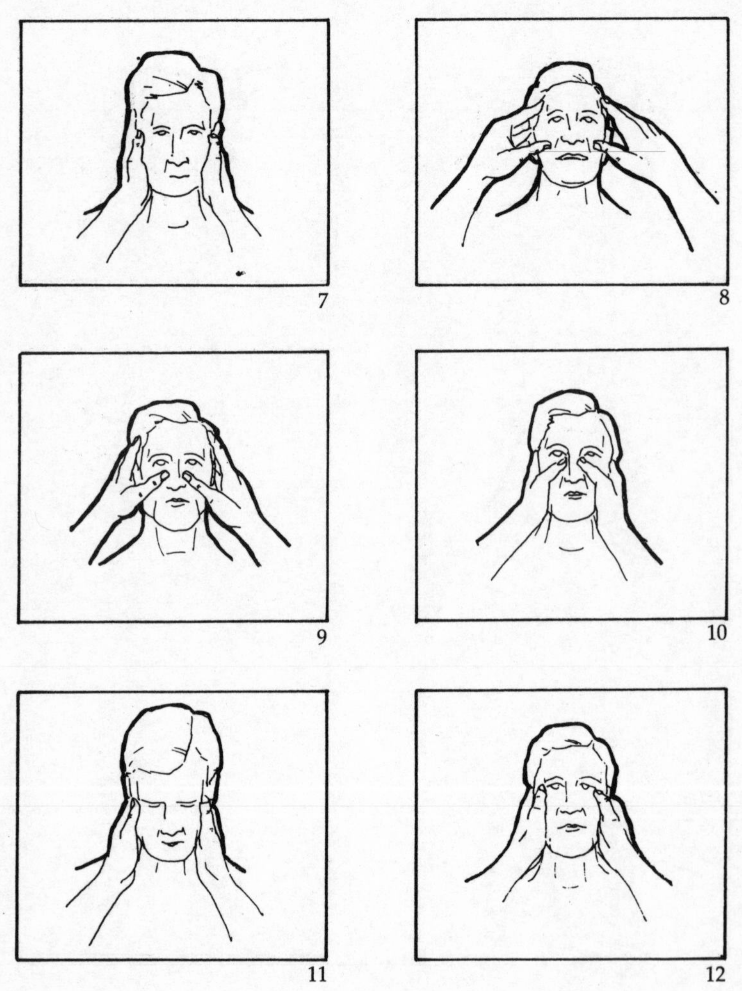
7
8
9
10
11
12

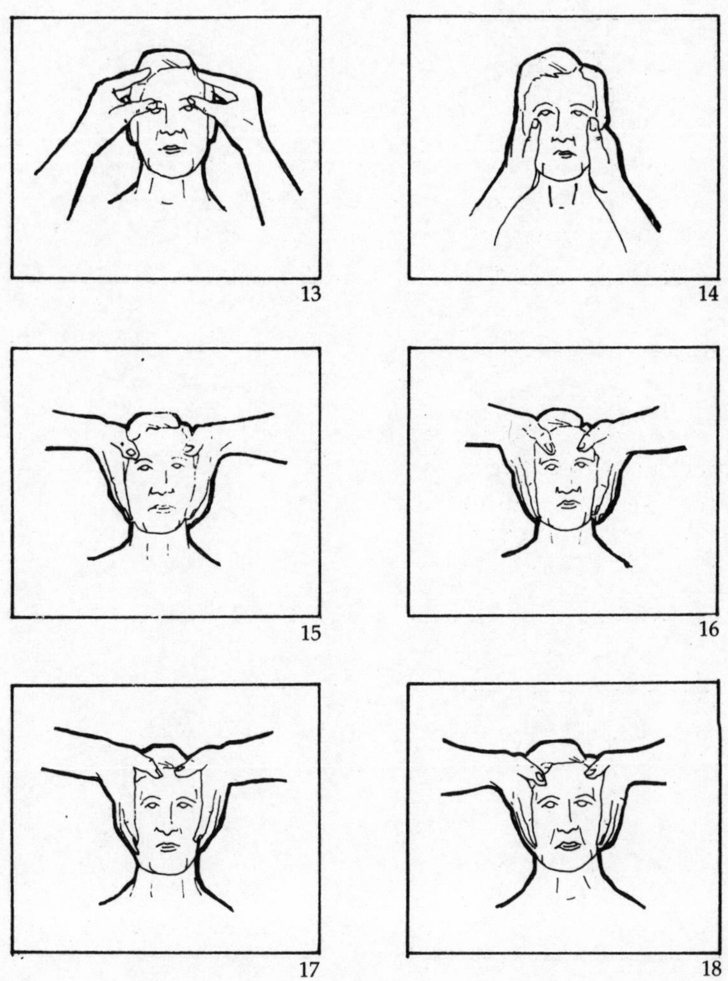

13 14 15 16 17 18

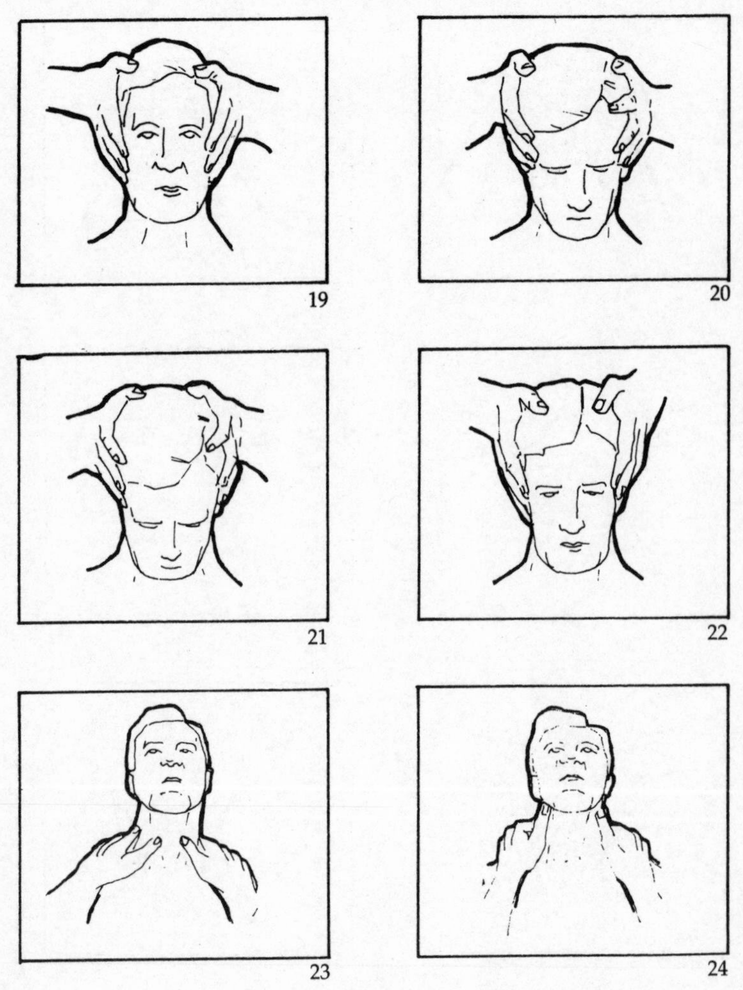
19
20
21
22
23
24

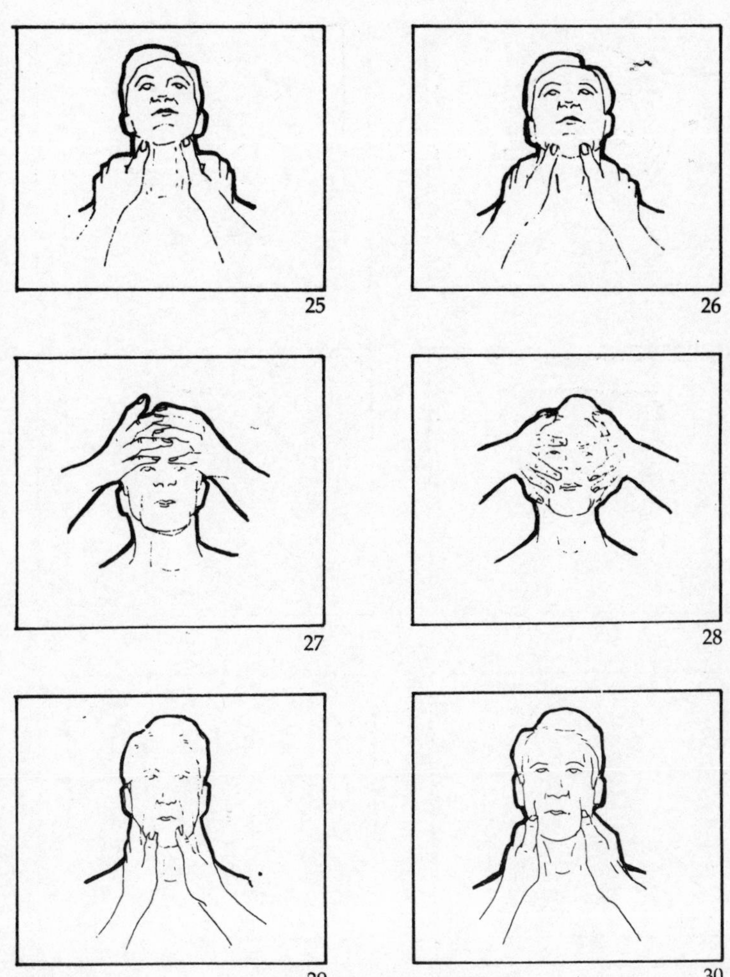

25 26 27 28 29 30

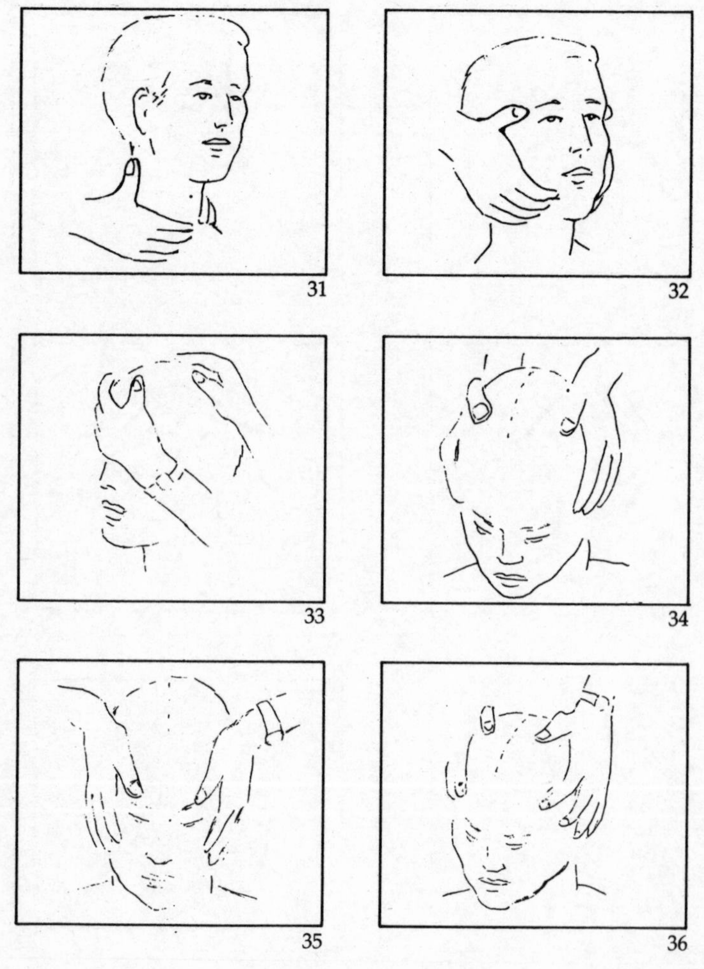
31
32
33
34
35
36

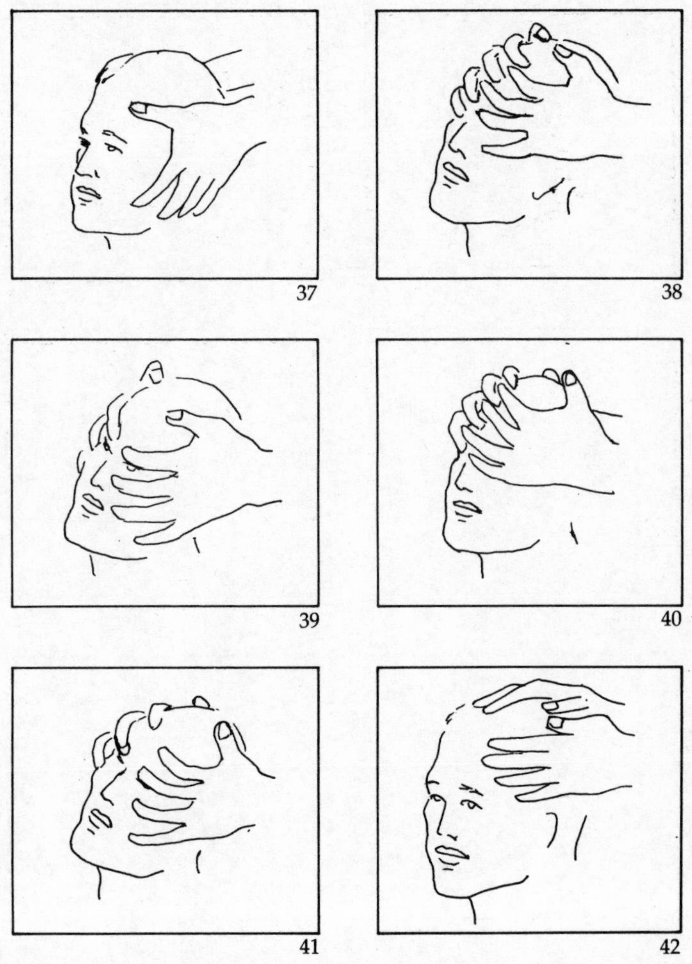
37
38
39
40
41
42

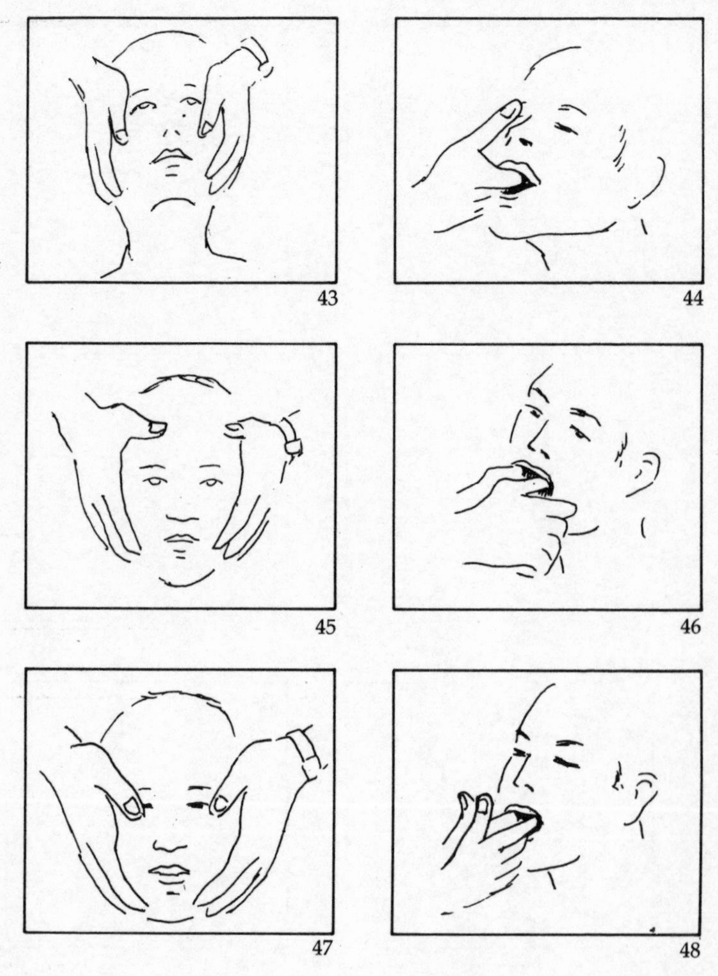
43
44
45
46
47
48

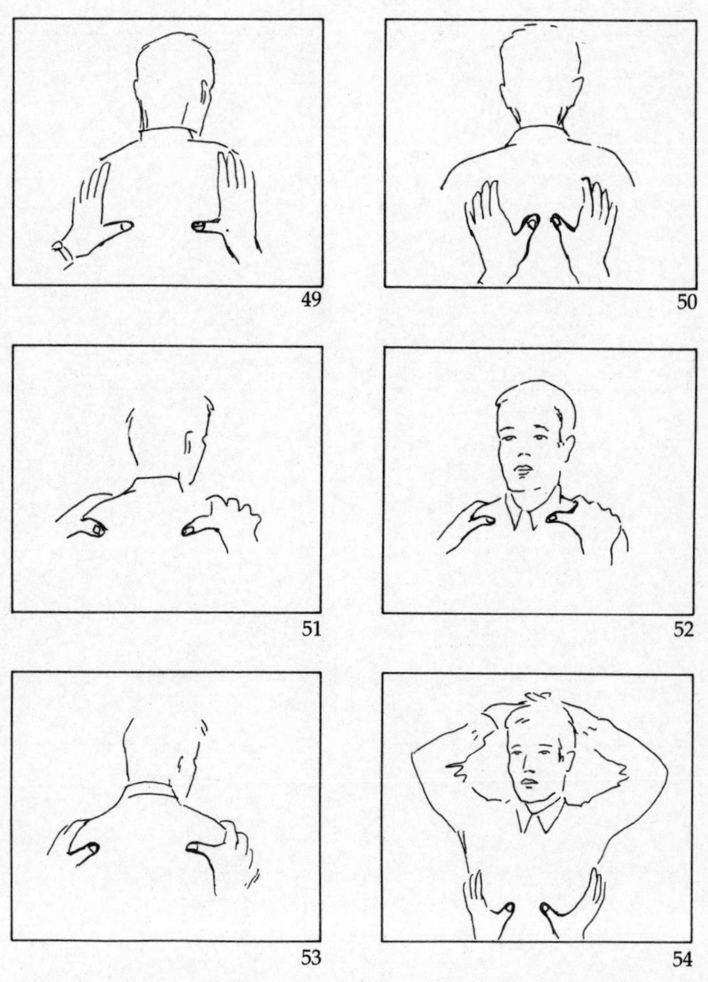
49
50
51
52
53
54

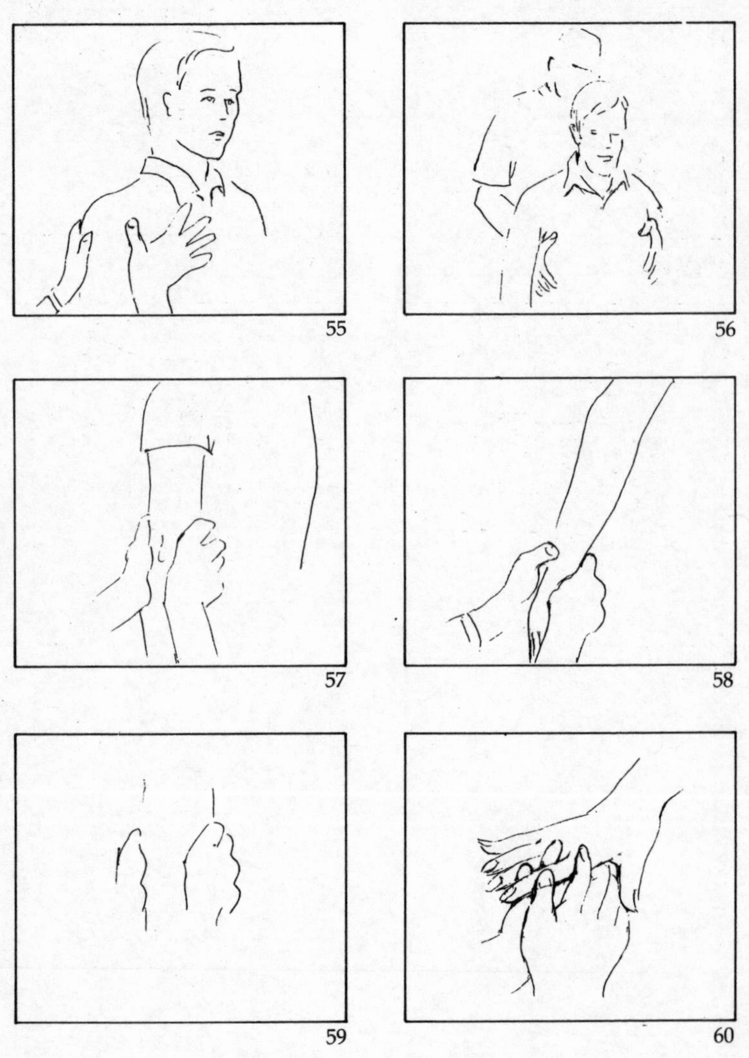
55
56
57
58
59
60

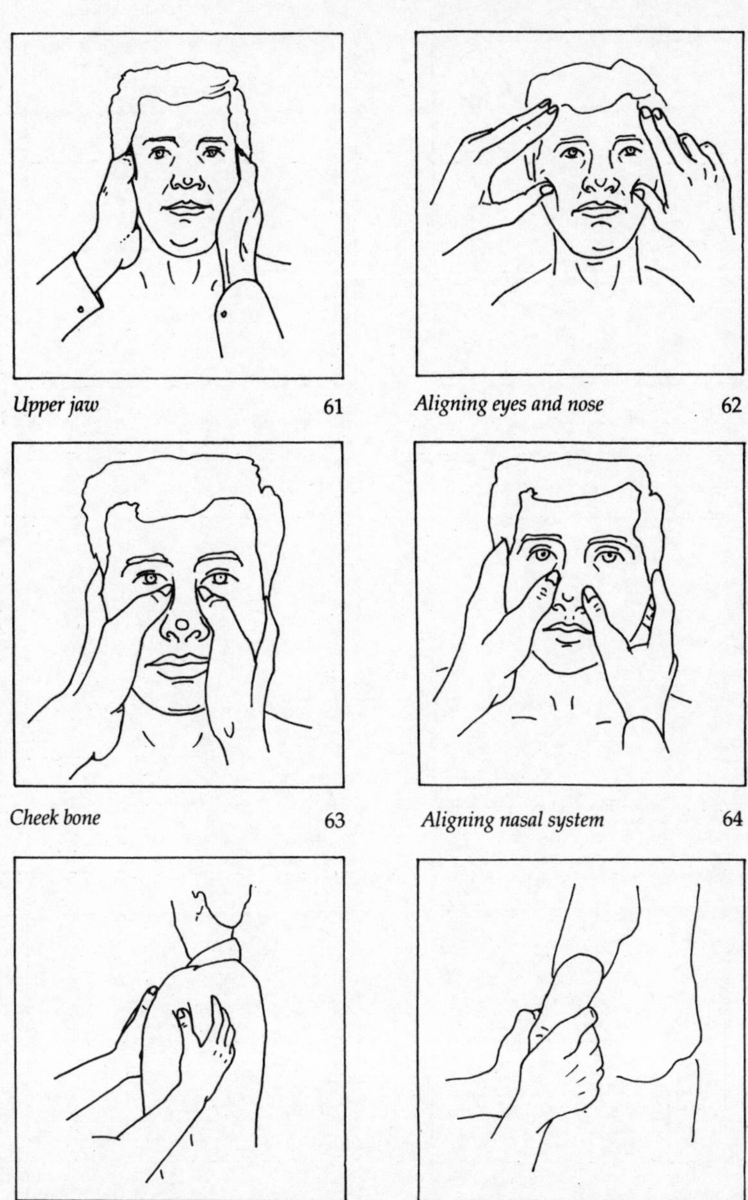

Upper jaw 61

Aligning eyes and nose 62

Cheek bone 63

Aligning nasal system 64

Aligning shoulder joint 65

Aligning elbow joint 66

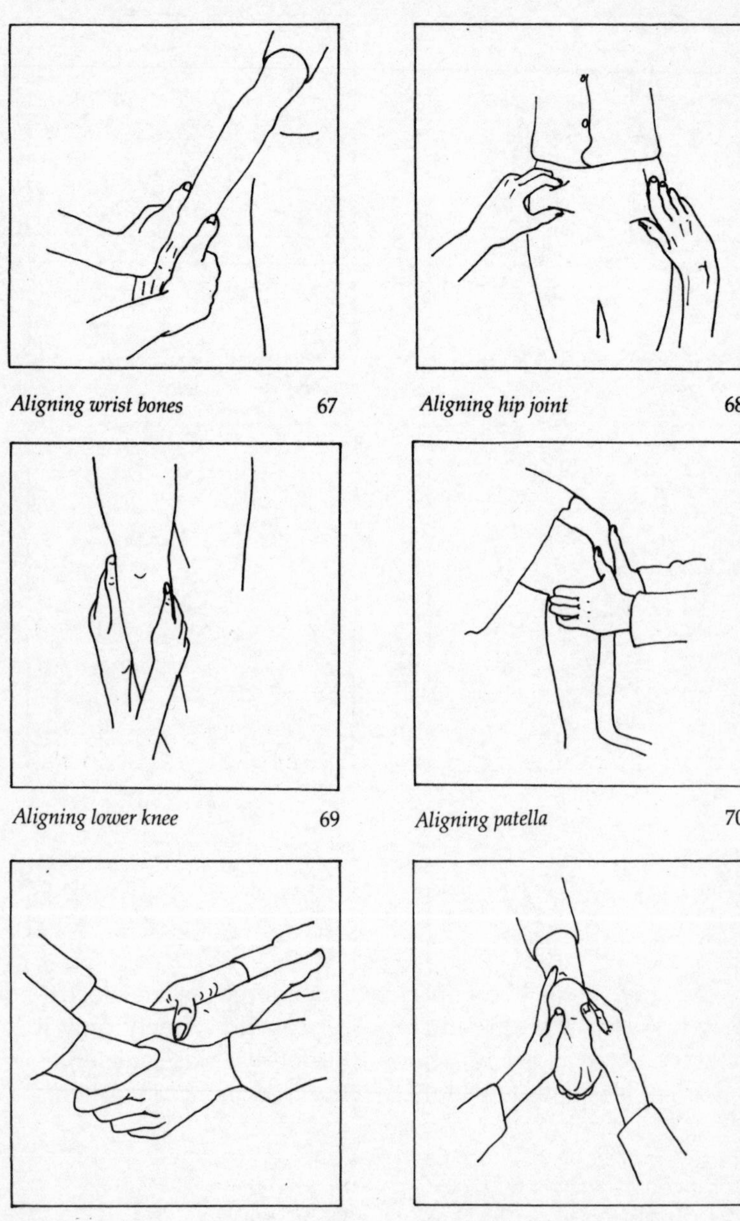

Aligning wrist bones 67

Aligning hip joint 68

Aligning lower knee 69

Aligning patella 70

Aligning ankle bones 71

Aligning heel bone 72

8

Energy in the Feet

WHEN ONE THINKS about general health, it is most unlikely that our thoughts would immediately include our feet; however, in the feet we find all the hormonal reflexes. In order to stimulate or relax the secretions of these hormonal glands, the manipulation of certain pressure points in the feet can be very useful. On my travels all over the world I have seen methods used that have been applied and tested by earlier civilisations and massage or palpations that serve to balance the energy in the human body.

Every gland and every organ in the body has a terminal nerve ending in the extremities — the feet, the fingers, and the face. The body may be considered as an electro-magnetic field through which power can flow freely only if the nerve endings are functioning properly. Massage serves to unblock and stimulate these nerve endings. This helps each gland and organ to function correctly.

Back in the sixties I was invited to visit some distant relatives of my wife who lived in a small village in Ayrshire, Scotland. The gentleman concerned had travelled throughout the world and at the end of our visit he handed me a little book, called *Stories The Feet Can Tell*, and extracted my promise that I would read it with an open mind and great attention. He had been telling me about things he had learned about using reflexes in the feet — in other words, what is now called reflexology — and I do not doubt that I must have appeared sceptical to his claims. I did read the book and went back to visit him again, because I wanted to hear all that he could tell me about this form of therapy. Since then I have followed the developments of reflexology with great interest. Some time after that first introduction I attended a medical conference where I met several people who lectured on the subject. In my work as an acupuncturist I obviously deal with pressure points and energy balance and therefore I followed these lectures with fascination.

Soon I realised that such methods greatly serve to stimulate the endocrine glands and that by massaging or palpating specific areas of the feet, somewhere in the body energy will result. The endocrine glands themselves have an energy — subject to vibration — and these glands represent balance in the body. As physical activity depends greatly on body energy, the endocrine glands clearly play a tremendous role, as we saw earlier.

However, before applying any pressure in a foot massage, in order to transform energy from the feet into balanced energy, one should always check first whether the feet are tender. If there is any tenderness in the feet, then gently comfort them before proceeding. Then, with the left hand under the foot and the right hand on top of it, relax for a while — for at least two minutes. This is a way to re-energise and it will make one feel considerably better. A good indication of this is the fact that after completing this exercise the pain of tender feet will mostly have disappeared. This simple exercise is in preparation for palpation with the thumbs of the different sensitive areas in the feet. You can do this yourself, but it is better if another person is willing to do it for you.

The secret of endocrine balancing is to bring into play the qualities of body energy. The best method is that in which one uses the thumb of each hand for the contact, the thumb being the most important part of the hand for polar energy. All individuals can help themselves, but it is also possible to help others to restore the endocrine balance. This method is also called zone therapy and the zones can reach the very important centres of life — the *shakras* — to improve the body energy balance. Great benefits can be obtained by using these simple manipulations.

It is most interesting that proof of the benefits of this particular method can be obtained by taking a Kirlian photograph. This method of photography, as we know, serves to show in black and white the energy outflow from the body, most especially in the extremities and facilitates our understanding of what is happening inside the body. The hands and feet give particularly good readings of the energy outflow.

I remember a while ago when my children were all home for a weekend and they decided to go for a long walk together along the beach. All four of my children are involved in the medical profession, two in conventional medicine and two in alternative medicine and they are always interested in some of the newer or more unusual methods being followed in my practice. My son-in-law, too, is a medical doctor and he especially always likes to discuss the pros and cons of such methods. I am sure that he had his own thoughts on Kirlian photography, but when they returned from their walk we were just in the process of tidying away the Kirlian photography equipment. They all confessed to being weary and my son-in-law suggested that I take a Kirlian photograph of his feet, as if to prove a point. Having done so, there was hardly any sign of energy outflow at all and I realised that he was slightly worried by this. The next morning I talked him into having another photograph taken and he was greatly surprised to see the difference. The later photograph showed a beautiful aura of energy and this quickly restored his confidence.

Like my son-in-law, I too was rather sceptical initially when I was given the book *Stories The Feet Can Tell* by my wife's relative, but I have since become convinced that these methods are of great value.

It would be useful if we could all go walking barefoot more often, if possible in the sand on the beach where we are forced to use the muscles in our feet to a much larger extent than when we are wearing shoes. We could even go barefoot in the snow. This may sound like a chilly experience, but I once spent Christmas and New Year in Switzerland and I was told by my hosts that it would bring good luck for the new year if I walked around the outside of the house in bare feet through the snow immediately after midnight on New Year's Eve. Well, on occasions like that one does not walk, let me assure you; it is more likely that one runs. However, we all took up the challenge and found it a most exhilarating experience. The feet tingle and one feels very much alive. As to the promise that it brings good luck, I am not too sure, but it certainly makes one feel good!

By all means let us give the reflexes of the feet a little bit of a push at times, because we tend to overlook the fact that we owe so much to them. Unfortunately, the feet are only appreciated when we are experiencing some problems with them. Chilblains are a sure sign that we have been pampering ourselves too much and have taken insufficient care of our feet. If you feel that walking barefoot in the snow is too drastic for comfort, you may decide to have a cold footbath instead. Another way to stimulate your feet and to help the reflexes is with gentle massage. This becomes a form of aromatherapy if you use some *Hypericum perforatum* oil and this ingredient is used in Dr Vogel's St John's Wort Oil. This may be an old-fashioned remedy, but let me assure you that it has a very beneficial effect on tired feet. A few drops of St John's Wort Oil may also be mixed with some lemon juice and you will soon feel the refreshing action of this combination.

I have already mentioned chilblains, but even with problems such as skin eruptions caused by ringworm, hot and cold footbaths are of great help. When snow stamping or walking barefoot, use some St John's Wort Oil for aftercare of the feet. It is also advisable to add some bicarbonate of soda to a hot footbath, or some thyme or hayflowers. You will soon discover how refreshing this can be.

In cases where foot problems occur as a result of circulatory difficulties, I can wholeheartedly recommend the following treatment, which I learned about in the Far East. This exercise should be done each morning after waking up and each night before retiring. Place a basin of cold water at the side of the bed and keep a towel handy. Before getting up in the morning place both feet into the water. After the count of ten move both feet from the basin on to the towel and dab them dry. Now exercise the toes as if trying to pick up a marble. Repeat this exercise between ten and thirty times. Before going to bed at night follow the same procedure and you will find that when you step into bed your feet will be glowing. The important thing to remember with this exercise is that it should be done for a minimum of sixty days if you wish to feel the full benefit. You may think that this exercise is too simple to be beneficial, but do not let its simplicity deceive you.

Good foot exercises and proper care of the feet are always important because the feet are really very good indicators of how the body feels as a whole. When people complain of tired feet this often means that somewhere in the body something is out of balance. The sooner that such signals are understood and heeded, the sooner this can be remedied. It really is quite something that certain reflexes in the feet can warn us that specific organs in the body are in danger and need attention. Once the reflexes in the feet have been studied, one can easily find out from these reflexes whether the cause of the problem lies in the liver, thyroid, kidneys or other organ.

All this goes to show how much our feet deserve our good care and attention. Do give them the occasional gentle massage or work on the reflexes by pressing the pressure points. Use some fragrant oil in a footbath and enjoy the relaxation that ensues. So often, the feet are regarded as ugly parts of our anatomy, yet what would we do without them? Like so many things, we will hardly appreciate them until they let us down. The balance of your body is totally reliant on your feet, as people who have been unfortunate enough to lose a foot will be able to tell you.

The feet also contain a wealth of acupuncture points as well as the pressure points that are so important for the endocrine system. Through these points we are able to influence the energy throughout the whole of the body, carrying it to the various glands and organs.

Much of the responsibility for our health rests on our own shoulders and it is in our own best interest to pay heed to these indicators. I often remind patients of the words of Dr Osler, a man with an admirable medical background: "When the nerves of the eyes and *feet* are properly understood, there will be less need for surgical intervention."

For quite some time now I have had the good fortune of being acquainted with a very knowledgeable person in the field of reflexology and aromatherapy — Shirley Price. I asked her about recent developments on these subjects and she was kind enough to share her thoughts with me.

You may know that karate is a Japanese system of self-defence, but perhaps you do not know the origin of the word: *Kara* means open, and *Te* means hand. Therefore karate means "open hand". You may wonder why I refer to karate in a book on energy and ways of balancing the body for the maintenance of good health? Because true karate is all about the balance of the mind and body in defence (not attack). True health is also about the balance of the mind and body in defence, against attack from bacteria and other harmful effects from the outside.

All natural therapies aim to keep the body in balance, naturally endeavouring to bring harmony between all the different bodily systems — and the mind. When you correct an imbalance good health will prevail once more.

Most people tend to want others to take responsibility for retaining their health, when in fact the balance is restored more quickly when patients take an active and therefore positive part in their recovery, both physically and mentally.

Actually the prime responsibility must always be with the patient, helped by expert guidance from the therapist. As far as aromatherapy treatments are concerned it is advisable that therapists give the client "homework" in one or both of the following forms:

—pure oils to inhale and/or put in the bath;
—mixed oils or lotions to apply to the face and/or body, not only to help the cause of the problem, but also to alleviate the symptoms that show and are therefore upsetting to the patient.

The body has its own natural inbuilt ability to heal itself and when it does need help, natural therapies together with a positive approach on the part of both therapist and patient can usually do the job without resorting to synthetic pills and tablets with their accompanying side-effects.

An interesting test was recently conducted in the field of conventional medicine. A group of people with the same problem were equally divided into two halves. One half saw a consultant who gave them positive encouragement, showing real interest in their problems and giving them a positive diagnosis and an optimistic forecast. The consultant for the second half had a more negative and disinterested approach. I don't need to tell you that a much higher rate of recovery was evident among the people in the first group.

During consultations (and this is so for all complementary therapists with whom I have come into contact), it always pays to get the patient actively involved. Aromatherapists, unless they have other specialised training in addition to that in aromatherapy, are not usually qualified to diagnose as such. Trained people use the reflexes of the feet and ask relevant questions to discover both the physical and mental state of the patient and, of course, they spend time listening, so that the emotional state of the whole person can be assessed. From the answers they are given, it is possible to deduce which oils will be most likely to revitalise the systems of the body which are out of balance.

Aromatherapy means the use of aromas from essential oils to help therapeutically to revitalise and strengthen the cellular tissues. It should be stressed that I am talking of *essential oils* here, as nowadays a few people trade in "aromatherapy oils", which have not always seen a pure unadulterated essential oil.

Only true essential oils which have been either distilled or expressed from the plant of the same name (having nothing added and nothing taken away) are used in true aromatherapy. The exceptions are two well-known absolutes, rose and jasmine (very expensive) and benzoin resin (quite *in*expensive). These three are not pure essential oils, as solvents are used in their extraction process, but they are used by most professional aromatherapists in mixes for application to the skin or use in the bath. (They should never be used internally.)

Each essential oil has the ability to help improve one or more system of the body, and many of the oils help to reduce what is commonly known as *stress,* in day-to-day living, or *depression,* which can occur as the result of anxious or stressful happenings.

Essential oils (like many other forms of complementary medicine) can restore energy, balance and harmony to a person's body rhythm when this has been interrupted by what is popularly called disease, i.e. they help to restore *ease* where there is *dis-ease*.

They can effect an improvement by themselves, for example when a person uses them in a simple home treatment in a fragrant bath for relaxation, following the guidance of a therapist or a specialist aromatherapy book. They can also be used in conjunction with many other complementary therapies such as osteopathy, acupuncture, remedial massage or skin treatments.

How is the use of essential oils different from using the whole plant? To answer that we need to know where in the plant the essential oil is to be found, and also to realise that its power is very concentrated. One drop of essential oil in 5 ml (a teaspoonful) of vegetable oil is sufficient to give the characteristic aroma of the plant.

Apart from expressed volatile oils, all of which are found in the skins of citrus fruits, essential oils can be found in the petals, leaves, seeds, stems, bark or roots of various plants, bushes or trees. They are present in very small amounts, locked in tiny oil "glands" which burst during distillation to release their precious oil.

When the whole plant is used, the concentration of healing power is necessarily spread over a greater area, so more plant material is needed to effect a similar result. Also, plants hold other healing properties in their structure which are made use of in herbal medicine. Aromatherapists use only the essential oils, which have quite a few advantages.

—They take up less space, so are much more convenient for travelling and holidays.
—They are ready for instant use, and will keep more or less indefinitely. The therapeutic qualities of some whole plants can change drastically after being stored for some time.
—The therapeutic effect is considerably magnified in the essential oil as opposed to the whole plant.
—They can be used in a greater variety of ways.

It is important to know that some plants contain more essential oil than others, so therefore the cost of essential oils varies immensely. It is also important to know that a true essential oil, without adulteration of any kind, is of necessity more expensive than an oil of the same name which has been "standardised", i.e. given a BP standard, which may even mean that alterations may have to be made to the natural oil to enable it to conform to what can be a lower standard than many plants are capable of producing.

Oils from plants grown free of any kind of pesticide and using only biological fertilisers are the most expensive of all. It is a debatable point as to whether they are significantly better than those to which non-harmful fertilisers and pesticides have been applied carefully and in the correct dosage. The former are still subject to acid rain, polluted air and ground water and the Chernobyl fall-out!

The most important points for a therapist to be sure of (until the essential oil trade for aromatherapy has been sorted out) are as follows:

—that no harmful chemical fertilisers or pesticides have been used (including those that produce quick lush growth, because just as forced strawberries have no flavour, the resulting oil is of a poorer quality);
—that he or she buys oils without the addition of alcool, nature-identical components, synthetic smell-alikes, or cheaper natural oils.

Pure essential oils are magical! Given true essential oils, the effects on the human body are amazing, and they can be used in many different ways to obtain the required therapeutic effects.

Their power is such that they should not be used in their concentrated form on the skin. There are a few exceptions to this rule, for example when treating burns and insect bites and other specific instances. In all other cases essential oils are always used in a carrier of some sort, i.e. anything neutral which carries the essential oil into the body.

A prime example of such a carrier is air, which carries essential oils into our noses when we inhale from a tissue. In fact, inhalation is one of the best ways, if not *the* best way, of using essential oils. Because our nasal passages have a direct line of contact with the brain, undiluted essential oils are put to work almost immediately to relieve problems like sudden stress, depression, headaches, respiratory disorders and insomnia.

Some of the oils which help these conditions are listed below.

Sudden stress:	basil, juniper, lavender, cedarwood, neroli, rose
Depression:	basil, bergamot, clary-sage, thyme, chamomile, camphor, geranium, lavender, frankincense, jasmine, neroli, patchouli, rose, sandalwood, ylang-ylang
Headaches:	lemon, eucalyptus, aniseed, chamomile, lavender
Asthma:	basil, cajuput, lemon, sage, thyme, aniseed, cypress, hyssop, lavender, marjoram, melissa, peppermint, pine, rosemary, savory, benzoin, clove, origanum
Sinus problems:	basil, eucalyptus, lemon, niaouli, lavender, peppermint, pine, clove
Insomnia:	basil, chamomile, camphor, juniper, lavender, marjoram, neroli, rose, sandalwood, ylang-ylang

Water is also a very useful carrier, especially when the oils are added to a warm bath. For all the above complaints (except asthma, as the hot water makes the oils evaporate too quickly and they are then too powerful for an asthmatic to cope with) plus general aches and pains, poor circulation, ongoing stress, arthritis, period problems and certain skin conditions, six to eight drops of the appropriate essential oils in the bath will produce amazing results in most cases.

Some oils that will help these additional conditions are listed below.

Aches and pains:	cajuput, coriander, caraway, eucalyptus, sage, thyme, black pepper, chamomile,

	camphor, juniper, lavender, marjoram, rosemary, clove, ginger, nutmeg, origanum
Poor circulation:	lemon, black pepper, camphor, cypress, juniper, rosemary, benzoin, rose, ginger
Ongoing stress:	basil, bergamot, clary-sage, petit-grain, thyme, chamomile, geranium, juniper, lavender, marjoram, melissa, benzoin, cedarwood, jasmine, patchouli, rose, sandalwood,
Painful periods:	cajuput, sage, aniseed, chamomile, cypress, juniper, marjoram, melissa, peppermint, rosemary, jasmine, tarragon
PMT:	lavender, melissa, neroli, rose, geranium, chamomile, clary-sage
Eczema:	sage, chamomile, hyssop, geranium, lavender, bergamot, juniper, sandalwood
Sore throat:	eucalyptus, thyme, cajuput, cedarwood, sandalwood, lemon, tea tree

Gargling is another way in which water can be used as a carrier for these natural oils and is invaluable in treating a sore throat or a cough. Put two or three drops of essential oil in half a cup of warm water and gargle with this to soothe and to kill off the infection (stirring before each mouthful as essential oils do not completely dissolve in water).

This is an appropriate place to make the point that essential oils in any carrier need to be used regularly in order to achieve the desired effect. Moreover, in cases of infection, their use should be continued beyond the "feeling better" stage, rather like a course of antibiotics, to ensure that the symptoms will not recur.

Compresses, again with water as the carrier, are most effective for localised problems such as arthritis, period problems, ulcers, athlete's foot, sprains and bruises; and for a bad head cold or catarrhal sinuses inhaling from a bowl of hot water and essential oils clears the head in minutes.

(Remember, however, hot water should not be used with essential oils for asthma.)

The last way of using essential oils with water as the carrier is, I think, an excellent one. It is possible to make tea using essential oils. If possible, tannin-free teabags should be used, though ordinary ones will do to make a very weak basic brew. If you have a stomach upset you may choose to put two drops of peppermint and one drop of fennel onto a teabag over which you pour one and a half pints of nearly boiling water. Stir well and remove the teabag. Then drink one cup of tea three times a day, saving the rest in a jug in the fridge until it is needed again.

It is great fun to make teas to help you go to sleep, teas to relieve stress, teas for reviving your brain (if you have a lot of work to do) and all from one packet of tea and a few little bottles!

One of the most popular methods of using essential oils is by application to the skin. Professional aromatherapists use a vegetable oil as their carrier so that they can carry out the special massage techniques now associated with aromatherapy. Shiatsu pressures, lymph drainage, neuro-muscular massage together with effleurage movements make up this form of massage, and it is one of the best and most pleasurable treatments that exists for dealing with stress and its associated problems.

A good well-trained aromatherapist will mix you a bottle of the oils that have been used in your treatment for your own use at home. You may be given them in their pure form for inhalation, baths or teas and perhaps also in a carrier oil or non-greasy lotion (the latter is much more pleasant to apply) for use after your bath or shower.

The skin responds very well to the application of essential oils in carrier oils, lotions or creams. A good quality aromatherapy skin-care range will rejuvenate the skin when used regularly, softening and smoothing its texture. People with problem skins, blocked sinuses, eczema, headaches, etc. can, with a specially formulated aromatherapy moisturising cream, take care of their skin at the same time as treating these problems. A hand lotion especially developed for arthritis softens the skin while at the same time relieves the pain and makes movement easier.

A new aromatherapy treatment developed by Shirley Price, called Swiss Reflex Therapy, is very similar to reflexology. It is now practised by quite a few aromatherapists, using essential oils. The patient takes an active part in the treatment, and is shown how to continue this at home, which may explain why it is proving so successful.

Swiss Reflex Therapy can be used in combination with an aromatherapy massage of the part of the body involved, or on its own where a massage would be difficult, contraindicated or unhelpful, for example if the part were swollen and painful. All the work on the feet is carried out to the pain threshold of each individual and the improvement is monitored by the patients themselves.

Aromatherapy is an amazing, delightful and rewarding therapy which fills anyone who embarks upon its study with never-ending enthusiasm. Because it is still in its infancy, being relatively new to this country, new facts are being discovered every day, and more research and attention is being given to the quality and the content of the essential oils used. Courses in aromatherapy are already getting longer, in order to accommodate the increasing amount of theory which needs to be taught. One day, no doubt, one will have to take a degree in something or other in order to practise aromatherapy. However, that may then prevent many caring people from being able to take it up as a career and doing much useful work to help the lives of themselves and others. The aspect which must not suffer in this thirst for more theoretical knowledge is the practical application; this must remain of prime importance, I believe, as aromatherapy is probably the only therapy which can be carried out in its simplest form by anyone and everyone who first steps onto this fascinating path of restoring one's energy.

9

Energy in Sound

IT HAPPENS EVERY now and then that I am consulted by patients who for some mysterious reason have lost the use of their voice. Usually this is the after-effect of a cold or flu, and occasionally it is due to other factors. That still leaves those who inexplicably lose their voice for a few days and then, without any evident cause, regain it. This can often recur at a later stage. Sometimes such conditions can be reversed with homoeopathic or herbal remedies or with Niacin. Finally, we are left with those patients who simply lose their voice because of lack of energy.

This last category of patients need a boost to the immune system and for this we sometimes prescribe Imuno-Strength from Nature's Best or treat them with relevant exercises. They will have to learn how to balance their own energies and treat themselves with some of the exercises mentioned in the chapter on energy in the hands (Chapter 6).

Every molecule and every atom in this universe — animate or inanimate — is in constant vibration and these vibrations are extremely powerful. That power is also present in the human voice, which is used to influence others as well as ourselves. That the power of the spoken word is not a contemporary realisation becomes apparent from the old proverb, "A soft answer turneth away wrath".

The human voice can be used disruptively, but also reassuringly. Therefore, if we use the energy in our voice constructively, we will produce positive action. The whole purpose of speech is to use the energy created by the voice as a means of influence during communication. I well remember the soothing voice of one of my staff members, a lady who worked in our relaxation department with my patients. In her instructions to the patients her voice seemed to exert a certain therapeutic power. It was not so much her choice of words, but the timbre of her voice with which she soothed our tense and stressed patients. This energy may not be immediately apparent in all of us, yet we all can use our voice to comfort others.

Over the years I have attended quite a few seminars given by the well-known Dr John Diamond MD. He is an authority on the subject of voice energy and maintains that if we are able to activate our thymus gland, we will be able to produce this life energy in our voice and transmit it to others. Musicians are able to produce this energy through their music, and they use their musical instruments as others use their voice — for communication. They succeed in expressing that life energy through their musical instruments and when they connect, this rapport will be shared with others.

Once a musician has mastered the secret of his instrument's voice, he is able to use it by communicating it to others. In fact, music is an essence of life and when one feels a bit down and depressed, one should try and sing a song. I remember when as a child one of us was a bit downhearted or looked a bit off-colour, my grandmother would tell us to sing a song and we would soon see that life was a bit brighter than before. And she was right. It is a fantastic remedy, sometimes so much more effective than any professional medical help. We can draw on this energy whenever we feel the need for it, because the vibrations of the physical act of singing travel through all the cells of our bodies. Singing changes our outlook on life and I have advised people with suicidal tendencies, when they feel circumstances crowding in on them, to go into a room on their own and sing out loud. Singing works like a bridge between the physical and mental areas of our bodies and reinforces our lines of thought to enable us to make clearer and more realistic decisions.

The human voice can be used in negative or positive ways and few of us can deny having seen the depleting effect when people accuse each other of being useless. Imagine the difference when one receives a word of praise or comfort. One's negative image will be reinforced by positive energy and a kind word has restored many a relationship before it has reached the brink of destruction. Communication is such a precious possession and the human voice is the instrument through which compassion can be communicated to those in pain or discomfort.

The human voice is one of the most versatile instruments that is given to mankind and many times it will have created new hope in people who were in despair or who had lost their confidence or self-respect. The human voice can create with a single word an energetic feeling of deep emotional sympathy to comfort the worried, anxious or depressed person.

The human voice can cause mountains to be moved and drive out negative thoughts. Figuratively speaking, such thoughts *are* insurmountable mountains, and yet a word of encouragement can change the whole situation even as it is spoken. Sometimes I have noticed when I have been talking to a negative or a depressed person that the blank and withdrawn eyes will suddenly register an expression of amazement. It would seem that either my tone of voice or the use of one particular word has struck a chord. The attention is captured and the whole attitude changes. That person becomes more receptive to treatment. How much truth and wisdom is contained in the biblical saying, "A word fitly spoken is like apples of gold in pictures of silver" (Proverbs 25: v 11).

On my travels I have listened with fascination to Tibetans, who appear to communicate by changes in the intonation of their spoken language. The meaning of the spoken word alters according to the vocal vibrations and their ability to make their voices vibrate or hum greatly impressed me.

In China I was taught that the three important factors in reaching a diagnosis were to look, listen and feel. Of course I listen attentively to a patient's story, even though it sometimes is rather garbled. I also listen carefully to the vibrations in the voice. I listen for an energy feedback in the voice, from which I partially draw my conclusions. This is the great power of the human voice. It is a tool which enables one to see through the outside facade into the mind of the patient. Harmony and symphony in a voice is symbolic of the endocrine system, which is expressed through the thoughts and voice.

One's own voice can be used to sooth and comfort oneself and I have often pointed out to patients that when they say their prayers or when they meditate they should speak out loud so that they can hear their own voice. Listen to what one is praying for and how the voice expresses the thoughts. Softly, this voice will come back and bring the harmony to one's life energies that is so necessary to produce the energy for one's daily responsibilities.

Train your voice to speak positively, practise using your voice by singing to yourself or to others. Think of the mother who sings a lullaby to her baby; her baby will be soothed, but the mother also will find comfort and harmony. The energy flow will increase. Sometimes we need to open the door to the within and this can be done with a positive voice; using positive words instigates positive actions. One can begin to speak and sing with a greater confidence when the voice is beginning to express and instil energy. Use the energy in your own voice and learn to listen for it in the voices of others.

I find it impossible not to be inspired by music. Unfortunately, according to statistics, the hearing of many youngsters is becoming impaired as a result of being subjected to loud disco music or being permanently plugged in to a personal cassette player. When I think of inspirational music I do not mean "heavy metal". It is, however, undeniable that this kind of music does stimulate the energy and in the United States psychologists have expressed serious concern about the number of teenagers committing suicide when under the influence of such music. Surely this confirms the fact that energy can be conveyed by music — albeit that in this case the energy is negative and has a detrimental and destructive effect.

Think how ritual or tribal music can drive the participants in rites or tribal dances into a hypnotic frenzy or trance, when they are subjected to forces outwith their control. As easily as music can instil fear, it can also inspire peace.

We live in an age in which loud music is fashionable for the younger generation, but could it be that this is their way of trying to escape from the pressures and tensions in their young lives? As the human voice, by its intonation or a spoken word, can influence us, so can the sound of a perfect note touch a chord and restore our life energy.

The earth has been called the womb of the solar system and here cosmic energy is at work. This natural energy will create a conducive atmosphere of harmony for negative and positive energies, expressed in a language we can understand and convey to others, if we consider ourselves part of that creation.

These natural forces are extremely powerful and can therefore be used as healing tools. Although we sometimes think of life energy as an intangible substance, we must recognise its healing and energising power, and that its inherent flow of energy is important if we are to avoid or overcome energy blockages in the body.

A lot of tension is self-inflicted, as we often take things for granted or are envious of those around us who appear to be better off. Let us be grateful for the gift of life and for the gift of our voice and let us use our voice to give thanks for the energy we receive, which in turn can be given by us to others.

After a seminar some time ago I was handed an envelope by a lady who has dedicated her life to helping others. On opening the envelope, I found inside the following poem, written by Evelyn Nolt:

The Glory that is Earth

Man tread softly on the Earth
What looks like dust
Is also the stuff of which galaxies are made.

The green of Earth's great trees and simple grasses
Is the same music played in red
Throughout our trunks and limbs . . .

O Earth, living, breathing, thinking Earth
On the day we treasure you
As you have treasured us
Humanness is born.

And throughout all Light
A Radiance leaps from star to star
Singing: A Son is born
HUMANITY.

10

Energy in Food

IT IS CERTAINLY not my intention to go into great detail about energy in food, as I intend to devote a separate book to that subject at a later date. What I do want to pinpoint here, however, are the negative and positive effects of the food we eat.

Nutrition has gone far beyond the art of feeding and, today, over-nutrition has become as much of a problem as malnutrition. What I want to touch upon is the electro-magnetic energy present in food, especially that related to the polarity of the body. It is of the utmost importance that we learn how to combine food, as food of equal energy value will neutralise or destroy energy. If we picture the body as an electro-magnetic machine we can perhaps understand that the normal function of cells must be on the positive side. The function can be slowed down or stopped entirely according to the kind of food we eat and therefore it is necessary to find the correct acid/alkaline balance combination, both to regulate digestion as well as to allow the distribution of nutrients to the cells.

The concept of energy in food is a relatively new branch in the field of nutrition, especially when we talk about electro-magnetic energy (as opposed to calories), which is vulnerable to destruction by over-cooking, exposure to polluted air, over-ripeness or poor combinations. We must therefore learn about maintaining the acid/alkaline balance and it is in this subject I always try to instruct my patients. We must attempt not only to buy our food when it is as fresh as possible, but also to eat it while it is still fresh. This gives us the kind of nutrition that is acceptable to the cells, encouraging them to renew and rebuild the cell tissues.

In previous chapters I have already emphasised the importance of amino acids for the effective digestion of protein that is essential if we are to maintain the human body in peak performance. As proteins must be changed into amino acids before they can be accepted as body builders, it is interesting to note that there are twenty-two known amino acids which are essential for our health, eight of which are indispensable. The energy obtained from amino acids is remarkable, as are the effects that will result from a change in dietary habits. It may surprise you to learn that such a step can inspire a major change of character in a person.

This is not an idle claim. I have seen clear proof of this in my work with prisoners, some of whom are criminals with life sentences. In this kind of research it is amazing to see how negative energies caused by an imbalanced food pattern can be transformed into a much more positive action. I have even seen a reversal in unwanted manifestations in hardened criminals with schizophrenic tendencies. The importance of using the right combinations to achieve positive energy from food should therefore receive the consideration it deserves.

Consider the problems we encounter because of "civilised" food. In this category fall all those foods grown with chemical fertilisers and "protected" by insecticides and pesticides, as well as foods processed with colourings and preservatives, i.e. convenience foods. Always check the contents of prepared food products by reading the labels carefully. Make yourself aware of the negative influences additives can have in terms of creating an imbalance between mind and body. It does not require a degree in nutrition to plan a balanced meal. It is mostly a matter of common sense. The golden rule is to keep food as fresh as possible. Also familiarise yourself with the value of using herbs for cooking, as this is a way of introducing a rich source of minerals and mineral salts into the system. This is relatively easy nowadays, considering the availability of fresh herbs. Not only are herbs of service to the digestive system, but your food will also be more tasteful and appetising.

Never lose sight of the fact that processed and pre-cooked foods have lost much of their nutritional value in the processing administrations.

For the sake of our health we require a wide range of vitamins, minerals and trace elements to produce energy. Health and energy are interdependent. Unfortunately, in an increasing number of newspaper and magazine articles we read about the amazing health-giving properties of particular foods or the incredible dangers of other foods. Such reports only serve to make us more confused. Some basic knowledge of nutrition together with a measure of common sense is all we need in order to be able to eat in a healthy manner.

Try to remember what it is like after spending a few days in bed because of a flu attack. Your arms and legs look thinner and your energy is at a low ebb. Yet the level of energy is quickly built up again when the diet contains adequate amounts of proteins and carbohydrates. The vital organs react speedily and gratefully to positive inputs.

It is commonly believed that for a quick boost of energy one should take a spoonful or a cube of white sugar. Let me tell you that a slice of wholemeal bread is an equally effective energy source. The idea that the glucose obtained from sucrose is absorbed more quickly into the bloodstream than the glucose that comes from bread or other sources of carbohydrates is based on a misconception. The difference in expediency of absorption is minimal — so small in fact that it is hardly noticeable. On the other hand, taking a spoonful of sugar for a quick "lift" too often carries with it the danger of addiction to sugar, possibly resulting in increased weight and creating long-term health hazards, due to the number of calories sugar contains. If one feels the need for something sweet rather than a piece of bread, it is better to take a spoonful of honey, which is a more natural product than white sugar. This will provide you with the desired uplift and energy boost, but you should still remember that it is not the quantity but the quality of the food that is significant. Remember, too, that honey has the same calorie count as sugar.

Respect the fact that the body is selective and always endeavours to produce better health. Unless we support it in the proper fashion, we will not be able to help it in its efforts to convert food into energy and, ultimately, health. We will degenerate and the signs and symptoms of this will then become evident in our daily life, manifesting themselves as diminished energy.

The correct food to eat is food that contains the basic requirements for energy and this will certainly not be found in, for example, a tin of tomato soup that has never even seen a tomato! When we eat the right food we can expect new tissue to be formed more quickly and as a result of improved eating habits —discontinuing our intake of "wrong" foods — we will also notice that an increased amount of energy will be obtained from a reduced food intake. This becomes especially clear when people change to a raw food diet largely based on organically grown food. The results they then experience can sometimes be beyond their expectations. Their health will improve and the skin will reflect the improvement of their internal health. They will become more alert and radiate energy. And, if we are honest, this can all be achieved by merely applying our common sense to our dietary habits.

Some time ago I attended a lecture given by a well-known immunologist. He stated quite categorically that there was no such thing as good food any more. I must admit that I tend to agree with him, because if our food has not been adulterated with chemicals during its cultivation, it has been exposed to negative energies from the polluted air that cannot be avoided. Fortunately, despite this factor, I am able to see what happens when patients change from a quantity diet to a quality diet. They report the disappearance of problems such as headaches, constipation, nervous tension and depression. In some cases they have lived with these complaints for so long that they have become a part of their existence. Often such problems are replaced by an energy which they have never experienced before. In the light of this I would advise everyone to try and eat organically grown food wherever possible. Even if this is not always possible in practice, please try to keep your food as fresh and natural as possible; use grains, vegetables, fruits and nuts, and your body will respond favourably.

We can see the difference even if more whole brown rice is introduced into the diet. This is an excellent energy-giving food, resulting in an improved yin and yang balance. Try a combination diet. There are so many ways in which we can improve the way we eat. Follow the laws of nature and keep your food simple in order to bring out this vital energy. Pay attention to the fats and oils you take. In this respect I can recommend the excellent book *Fats that Cure and Fats that Kill*, written by Udo Erasmus.

Life and energy are inseparable and it is a well-known fact that all living things need energy from one source or another, because life cannot continue without energy. Food is our main source of energy and therefore we have it in our power to exert a favourable influence, which is much more preferable than continuing in our detrimental ways.

I love to write about food as a living energy. We may not be aware of it, but a simple potato retains about 30 per cent of the original energy received from sunlight. On the other hand, beef only gives us 4 per cent. An acre of land can produce in a year almost nine times as much potato protein as beef protein. There are many misconceptions and much ignorance about these aspects of the food we eat.

Another fact is that proteins are certainly necessary for the human body, but let us look at the many underprivileged people in the world and consider their low intake of protein. Because they — mostly unknowingly — use the right source of protein, they probably have much more energy than if they were to consume the same amount of dead protein as we do in our part of the world.

It is essential that we realise that there is no substitute for protein; however, protein has to provide all the material required to build body tissue and body fluids, we should also understand that it needs to be the right kind of protein. Most of us were probably taught at school that meat and fish provide us with first-class protein. To a naturopath, however, the best sources of protein are to be found in foods such as vegetables, fruits, nuts, soya and grains. Moreover, it is just a fairytale that carbohydrates are fattening. This is not the case if there is a good balance between carbohydrates and protein. Complex carbohydrates, of which we need very little, will not make us fat. On the contrary, they will give us energy and act as a good balance.

On my many travels throughout the world it always hurts me to see, especially in Eastern countries, how the people living in countries where rice was once the staple diet have grown used to our negative energy-giving food. Thinking of the health problems they are struggling with nowadays, I cannot fail to feel ashamed that in a way we are responsible for the damage those people are inflicting on their health. We have introduced them to such negative foods as fizzy drinks full of chemical additives and artificial colourings, and convenience foods.

Everyone needs a healthy diet, but is there such a thing? One can really not establish a single ideal diet, as dietary requirements will differ very much from one person to another. We can, however, use our common sense and decide to eat healthy food in the knowledge that it will give us energy. I do not aim to turn us all into vegetarians, but I have seen many times that when a patient has adopted a vegetarian diet, largely based on raw foods, how he or she has thrived and obtained the best results one could wish for.

However, I will always advise any patient, if he or she prefers not to abstain from meat, never to touch any meat coming from the pig. Bacon, ham, gammon and pork sausages are all dead foods because of the eating habits of the pig, and often do more harm than good due to their high acid and animal fat contents. Another warning I would give is that if food is not to be eaten raw, then conventional cooking methods are preferable to cooking food in a microwave oven, which is more likely to lead to further problems. It is always better to cook food in a casserole, a pressure cooker or a steamer.

Always remember that foods that are rich in vitamins, minerals and trace elements are indispensable in a good diet. It saddens me to learn that only 2 per cent of the British population have good, healthy teeth. If we look at the inhabitants of underprivileged countries, and especially at those living in some of the South Sea islands, we will see that their older generations often still have beautiful teeth. When we think of the way they live, we can only conclude that instinctively they must know what is the right kind of food for them — and this is often evident in their physical beauty.

In the western world so many people have even lost their ability to digest or absorb raw foods. From childhood they have been filling their stomachs with all the wrong food and in order to give their stomachs a chance again, they must learn how to satisfy themselves with responsible food. It is time we took stock and adopted a positive mental attitude to our diet. Because the functioning of the body depends on the food we eat, the expression *"we are what we eat"* contains a lot of truth. Tests have been conducted in which rats were fed on a variety of foods, from which it was concluded that even rats would not be able to survive on the food on which we feed ourselves. This is largely because that food has no sustaining nourishment; indeed, sometimes the additives act more like a poison than as a source of energy.

Let us look at the whole food question with some intelligence and common sense. We will then understand that only by eating a balanced diet of good natural food will we receive the nutritional value we need to produce the necessary energy. It is a fact that we feel more energetic after a fast. For a relatively short period of time we may decide to survive on fruit juices only. This serves to cleanse the body and gives it a chance to rid itself of some of its toxicity. Few of us are prepared to admit that we consume far more food than is actually required. Even for a common cold, a headache or a stomach problem, fasting can prove effective and we will feel much more energetic even after having fasted for a short while. Who wants to feel half alive when they could be healthy and energetic and able to enjoy their life to the full?

There is another matter concerning food that is relevant here. We must ask ourselves why there is so much talk about allergies and viruses at present. I promise you that in most cases we need look no further than the average diet, which certainly does not help the immune system to do its work effectively. Only by using energy-giving food can we encourage our immune system to withstand the attacks on our health stemming from interference with our food, water and air, the three things which are, or should be, the main sources of energy.

I find it most encouraging that our government as well as the British Medical Association are now investigating the effects on human health of the hidden dangers in pesticides, insecticides and fertilisers. This area of research also includes the use of preservatives and colourings and more and more information in this field is being released to the public. It is no myth that ingesting increasingly high doses of chemicals has been found to be harmful. This could well be a causative or contributory factor in cancer, liver damage and certain nervous disorders. It also appears that irradiation of food will enhance the toxicity of pesticide residues.

To me, it is equally frightening to learn that fluoride and sulphides can cause allergic reactions in acute asthma sufferers. Even a simple allergy should not be allowed to go unchecked, because only too often we learn that serious problems were triggered initially by a simple allergy. In my book *Viruses, Allergies and the Immune System* you can find plenty of evidence to back up such claims.

Above all, let us not forget that all diseases begin with a loss of energy and that we should resort to all available methods in order to achieve or restore a balanced flow of energy. We do not actually live by the food we eat, but we live by the energy created by that food. Deficiencies may necessitate the use of food supplements, but always look first at your dietary regime to see if that is where the fault can be found and corrected.

It is sad to consider that it cannot be much more than fifty years since food was grown without chemical interference and therefore contained all the required nutrients. Today, most of the soil's supply of minerals and trace elements has been depleted; therefore the nutritional value of the food grown in it is inferior.

Do you not think it sad when a vegetable has lost the rich individual smell and colour it once had? You can rest assured that it will also have lost its vital energy. Nature contains a boundless supply of energy if we would take the bother to learn where to find it. Every single cell in the human body will make contact with every molecule of food we consume. If that food has positive energy, it will result in positive energetic action.

We use our brain for lots of ineffectual and unimportant purposes, but let us train ourselves instead to concentrate on what we eat. I am glad to say that, fortunately, dieticians are also beginning to think along these lines. I am convinced that more knowledge is still to be discovered on essential nutrition. We will learn that nutrients work together as a team in the science of energy. If we lack energy, always remember to look at several factors. Do we eat the correct food? Do we drink sufficient amounts, and the right kind, of fluid? Do we take enough exercise? It is sometimes surprising when, combatting deficiencies, we see how quickly our bodies react. Sometimes we see this with muscle weakness, by giving a little of Nature's Best B-Complex. Or, as I recently saw with a patient, who, from a dwindling overweight person, regained so much energy, as the fat-burning mechanism, which is an important part of the ability to keep working, was lacking in L-Carnitine and amino acid lysine — which can be made by the body, given sufficient vitamin C, B vitamins and iron. For keeping slim, healthy and energetic, this supplement can prove vital. Athletes find that they exercise better when they are diet-conscious and use these supplements. Let us remember that life can be very sweet indeed if our bodies are a field of vital energy!

Conclusion

THAT WONDERFUL WORD "energy" conveys hope for the future, even though with our present knowledge we can only scrape the surface of what it signifies. The future of medicine may well lie in positive energy, although we also know that energy can be used to effect the destruction of mankind. If for no other reason than that, we must face up to the problems that energy has created in the barren and desolate areas of Hiroshima and Chernobyl. We should also consider the reported increase in the incidence of cancer and leukaemia near nuclear power stations and the geopathic stress of electro-magnetic fields. We have to learn to use energy to our advantage and in doing so to exercise great care. If we neglect to do this, energy could destroy us all and wipe mankind off the face of the earth.

Are we reaching the stage where life today is a case of survival of the fittest? Are we paying due care and attention to our natural immunity? Do we exhibit that vital energy that man is supposed to have, or do we now employ energy only to wipe out plants, animals and even mankind?

Patients sometimes exhibit signs of unnaturally high levels of radium that can only suggest the influence of radiation. Similarly, the presence of strong energies such as those exerted by silicone, germanium and magnetite in soil samples spells great danger. In our part of the world the after-effects of the Chernobyl disaster can also be observed.

Unstable energy influences may lead to simple allergic reactions and expose the weaker immune system to prowling invaders. Major problems can be the result, such as ME — the post-viral syndrome. It does not stop there, as many degenerative diseases can progress beyond the stage where help can be given. Again in relation to Chernobyl, a Moscow newspaper reported recently that the number of deformed animals born on a Ukrainian farm more than thirty miles from the disaster area has created a great fear in the people living in the area.

There is no doubt that our environment needs cleaning up. Only by a positive and concentrated move towards improvement in the quality of individual ideals, conditions and actions can this be brought about. Positive thoughts or vibrations cannot fail to produce positive results. Pay heed to your inner voice, conscience and senses of taste and smell. Do you have stomach pains or a bloated feeling after eating a meal? Do you have tooth decay? Do you feel like a nap after your meal? Are you unusually tired and lacking in energy? Then there could well be a problem in the balance between positive and negative energy — the yin and yang balance.

It is this energy balance that dictates to our bodies. It is this same energy balance that helps us to digest food and determines whether our bodies gain or lose energy. Perhaps our living circumstances are not what they should be. Perhaps our food is not as natural as it could be. It is worse still if our food is depolarised through radiation or irradiation. Some governments have consciously permitted the radiation of perishable foods for the sole purpose of killing bacteria, insects and fungi, and increasing their shelf life. Do not forget, however, that irradiation does not differentiate between good and bad bacteria. Some of the problems today stem from the fact that "friendly" bacteria are being destroyed in such processes. It is unfortunate that one appears unaware of the old homoeopathic principle that one cannot set about destroying the bad without destroying some of the good.

All this is probably the deadly price we pay for today's incomplete knowledge of energy. That is why we have been hearing so much lately about viruses, parasites and bacteria. It is also the reason why salmonella has become such a familiar word. All these factors amount to a less effective immune system — the indicator of vital energy in man. Add to that the radiation dangers of the visual display units and geopathic stress. Still we have this great power within us, the innate energy and the mind energy, with which we can combat and overcome health problems. No matter how complex the problems, we can release this energy to help by reducing the stress factor.

The last thing I want to do is to paint too grim a picture of today's environment. Rather, I want to emphasise that with a positive mind we can reactivate that innate energy. Let me remind you of what I was taught in China: to look, listen and feel.

—First we look, and then we may hopefully find where we might have gone wrong. Look with a positive mind at the cosmic energy that envelops us and passes right through us and back again. A balanced energy flow suffers no blockage or interference.

—Then we listen. Yes, listen to good positive advice. Listen to the inner voice of our conscience telling us where energy could be disturbed and where it could possibly be adjusted. We listen for vibrations of energy, reminding ourselves of the fact that all energy is vibration and all vibration is energy.

—Lastly we feel. Use those hands that God has endowed us with in Creation. The hands can direct energies positively. Use the hands to balance energy in the knowledge that they are instruments of healing.

Health problems occur because of an imbalance in the poles, creating tension. Using zinc or copper magnets the balance between the north and south pole energies can be restored. After all, every organ, gland, muscle, tissue, bone or cell in the body has a direct or indirect connection with the surface of the body. Accept the fact that in the many nerve centres found on the surface of the human body, universal energy can be utilised to bring about a better health balance.

So often the treatment and advice referred to in this book have suffered from the reputation of being mysteriously linked to ancient secrets. I hope the reader will now understand that the correct explanation is to be found in maintaining a balanced energy. That previous civilisations were more aware of that aspect than our present society can most logically be ascribed to an intuitive intelligence. Accept it as a gift from our Creator and be grateful that you are a minute part of this great universe.

Bibliography

Allan, Leonard, Dr Ac. — *Painless Pain Control*, Allan, Margate, UK.

Davies, Paul, — *Super Force*, Unwin Paperbacks, London, Boston, Sydney.

Diamond, John, MD — *Life Energy*, Dodd, Mead & Company New York, USA.

Evans, Elizabeth, Dr — *Diet and Nutrition*, Octopus Books Limited, London, UK.

Hamaker, John D., — *The Survival of Civilisation*, Hamaker-Weaver Publishers, Michigan, California, USA.

Kaye, Anna and Matchan, Don C. — *Mirror of the Body*, Strawberry Hill Press, San Francisco, USA.

Maltz, Maxwell, MD, FICS — *Psycho-Cybernetics*, Melvin Powers Company, Hollywood, USA.

Parcells, Hazel — *The Electro-Magnetic Energy in Foods*, Parxcell School of Scientific Nutrition, Albuquerque, New Mexico.

Thie, John F. — *Touch for Health*.

Ullman, Dana — *Homoeopathy — Medicine for the 21st Century*, Thorsons Publishing Group, Wellingborough, UK.

Vogel, Albert, *Swiss Nature Doctor*, A. Vogel Verlag, Teufen, Switzerland.

Useful Addresses

Bioforce (UK) Limited
South Nelson Industrial Estate,
Cramlington, Northumberland NE23 9HL

Nature's Best
Freepost PO Box 1, Tunbridge Wells TN2 3EQ

Auchenkyle
Southwoods Road, Troon, Ayrshire KA10 7EL
Tel. 0292 311414

Culzean Castle Herb Gardens
Culzean, Maybole, Ayrshire KA19 8LE

Shirley Price Aromatherapy
Wesley House, Stockwell Head,
Hinckley, Leicestershire LE10 1RD